— NOT YOUR AVERAGE —

Recovery Book

Permission To Eat

A practical guide to
working yourself out of an eating disorder
during college, while celebrating
the awesomeness that is you!

——————— B Y ———————

LIBBY PARKER, MS, RD

Publishing Services provided by Paper Raven Books

Printed in the United States of America

First Printing, 2019

Paperback ISBN= 978-1-7338207-0-7
Hardback ISBN= 978-1-7338207-1-4

Table of Contents

Dedication

To all the foods that I avoided, but secretly wanted.
This is for you.

Introduction

Dear Reader,

You may be wondering why you picked this particular book off the shelf (or Amazon listing) when there are hundreds of other recovery books available. Well, my hope is to share with you what I wish I had known in college about treating my body right.

Let me begin by telling you about my first year in college. First time away from home and I move straight into the roommate-from-hell scenario. This girl was the anti-me. From our first email—where she told me that she didn't like doing laundry so she bought new clothes instead—to actually living with her, and her mess, and her loud hair straightening (have you ever heard someone slap the ceramic plates together with every stroke? It's sooo annoying!), I grew more pessimistic by the day.

She was a night-party person, I was a morning person with 8AM classes. She had her boyfriend and loud friends over at night when I wanted to sleep, shower, or just have some quiet time.

We lasted less than four weeks.

In the time we were stuck together, I spent as much time out of the room as possible. Prior to college, I had never been much of an athlete and had just started losing weight during senior year of high school due to—at the time—smarter health choices, like swapping a row of Oreos for an apple. Well, turn on the triggers of living away from home for the first time with a roommate who was making me seriously sleep deprived, and my need to control my environment amplified.

Getting out of the room in a small town in Wisconsin meant you could see everything in less than an hour. I began taking long walks through the scenic paths next to the creek and farms, earbuds in, listening to music. I was walking one, two hours, sometimes longer. Faster and faster. My thinning arms pumping away in a power walk to the beat of early 2000s music. Slowly, I began adding in short jog spurts. This would turn into running later in college, and eventually racing.

Once my roommate and I were separated (huzzah!), I was able to refocus on my studies, my friends, and my food. I'd recently discovered calorie counting from the countless women's magazines that were available at home, in line at the store, and in every waiting room. They said you needed to be aware of calories to lose weight, so I was. Somewhere along the line, I read about not going too low, so I made sure to stay in a range that wasn't "too" low (plus I liked food, I couldn't completely give it up).

Over the course of about two years, I dropped quite a bit of weight. At some point, I began meticulously recording my weight every few days with the scale that lived under my desk in the dorm.

I had no idea this was not healthy.

I mean, we're fighting the obesity epidemic! Weight loss is to be celebrated! I can lose weight. Not only lose it but also keep it off. I was a frickin' weight loss unicorn!

That first semester of college, I became aware of a career called "Registered Dietitian," which I think I read about in some women's magazine as someone helping people lose weight. A job helping people lose weight? I'm good at that. Sign me up!

So, I went to my career counselor and set about switching majors (I was pre-veterinarian, originally). I had to switch schools and pick up a minor and another year of school to make this transition because of all of the science I needed for nutrition (which was ultimately so helpful to my mindset with food; though it's not for everyone who majors in nutrition). While I slogged through cell and molecular biology, I rigidly counted calories, noting every morsel, to the point that I would eat just ¼ of a piece of Dove chocolate (those tiny ones that come in the big bag), and wrap up the rest for later. I was starting to over-exercise, telling everyone I was a "kinesthetic learner" to justify my habits of walking around the student center with my textbook and reading notes on the elliptical for hours.

My story has a happy ending (well, middle; I'm not done living yet!). Through the nutrition curriculum and wonderful professors teaching me that food is just food (and, no, sugar is not evil), and how our body uses food for every cell process (oh, Krebs cycle); along with friends and family cooking for me (thus not knowing what was in my food) and not wanting to disappoint them, I eventually stopped calorie counting and was able to slowly recover. It wasn't until years later that I was able to see what a mess I had been and that I had suffered from "atypical anorexia."

I couldn't see it while I was drowning in the disorder. In fact, I vehemently denied having problems, as many of my clients do. Today, I have gained that weight back and am happier than I ever was. I can't remember the last time I counted calories or wouldn't let myself have food that looked good. I don't binge. I can eat at any restaurant I want. Even better, I have learned how to communicate this to my clients and have helped hundreds of people, mostly college students, move towards peace with food and with their bodies.

I'm writing this to let you know that I understand what's going through your mind. The calorie counter that won't turn off. A headache that comes from not having "healthy" food at a party. The constant worry that others are judging my plate, my body, me. Worry about the binge that I think I will be able to control *this* time. The drive to see how far I can take it.

I don't wish that life for you.

The more I study the science of the body and what it does for us, the more I am in total awe and the more I feel completely at ease around food. Our bodies will take care of us if we let them. We don't have to think about making our heart beat, ensuring our lungs breathe, or that our kidneys filter fluids to produce urine. Our body does that automatically. The food we eat gets turned into muscle, bone, hormones, brain matter, saliva, and everything else in our body.

Your body wants to be in harmony with your mind. I'm here to help you find peace with food, and teach you what I wish I knew back then. I want to give you permission to eat.

Are you ready to make peace with food?

Turn the page and let's get started.

How To Use This Book

This book is meant to be a guide to help you recover from or prevent the development of an eating disorder. My goal is to empower and encourage you to live your best life in the body you were designed to have, not what society says you "should" have. I want you to be able to love yourself just as you are because you are truly worthy of love and acceptance.

You can read this book in one weekend and go back to relevant sections to take action. Or you can move through chapter by chapter, using the "take action" tips at the end of each one. While I wrote this book for college students, the information and tips can apply to those at any age. With my slowly-expanding knowledge on the subject, my goal was to make this gender-inclusive; however, it is limited by scientific research that does not include all genders.

For best results, I encourage you to keep a journal while you work through this book. At the end of each chapter, I ask questions that will build on each other, and it will be useful to look back on what you were thinking and see how that can grow and change.

Bonuses: Throughout the book, you will see this icon ★. This means that there is an accompanying worksheet or other online bonus available when you log into: **https:// learn-with-libby.teachable.com/p/permission-to-eat.** (If for some reason the link is not working, please email: info@ notyouraveragenutritionist.com.) This content is copyright of Libby Parker, and is for personal use only.

Chapter 1

My ED Ate My Homework

"The human body is about 70% water. So we're basically cucumbers with anxiety."
—Unknown

This is not a diet book.

This is a book for freeing yourself from the power food has over you. It will help you manage your relationship with food, so you can get on with the more important parts of life.

Before we dig in, I want to ask you a few questions. Take your time with these.

- What would it be like to feel confident and sexy in your current body?

- What would it mean for your life if you felt empowered and had higher self-esteem?
- What if your self-worth wasn't tied to your body or food choices?

I've been working with those with eating disorders for many years now and have found my passion specializing in helping college students cultivate healthy relationships with food and their body. While eating disorders do not discriminate (they occur in people of all sizes, races, gender identities, sexual orientations, locations, socioeconomic status, and at any age), most begin around puberty or early adulthood, especially during high school and college years.

Why is this?

Well, any time there is a big transition or stressor in life, people with a predisposition to developing an eating disorder are more likely to have the behaviors come out as a way of coping with the stress or worries of the unknown.

An eating disorder develops when someone uses food as a way to cope. Eating disorders are a way of coping with not wanting to feel emotions or deal with certain situations. They allow the person to become numb or focused on something else, in much the same way that someone would misuse drugs or alcohol. Eating disorders are not an addiction, though they can sure feel like it at times.

Eating disorders (EDs, for short) have both genetic and environmental components. This means you need the genes for an eating disorder to develop, but it won't be expressed without an environmental trigger. Some people can have the genes for an ED and go through their entire lives without seeing it expressed.

As ED expert Dr. Walter Kaye puts it, "Genetics load the gun, and environment pulls the trigger." In other words, a person can have the genes to develop an eating disorder but never express the thoughts or behaviors if there is no reason to use them to cope. Another person could have the perfect storm of trauma and environmental triggers but, without the genes for the ED, won't develop one.

Let's get specific. Why is college, in particular, such a big time for EDs?

Well, there are four things I've come to realize:

1. College is a major life transition, especially if the person is living away from home for the first time. College students may feel out of control with all the changes happening in their lives, and their food choices may seem like the only thing they have control over; *and* for the first time, they have complete autonomy about what foods they choose to buy instead of whatever was at home or put in front of them.

2. College age comes shortly after puberty, hence a normal time for ED development. During this time, hormones and body changes can leave people feeling like they don't belong in their own body. This is even harder on people who are misgendered by others (trans/gender-fluid/nonbinary). Developmentally speaking, this stage following puberty is very egocentric ("me, me, me"), making people believe that everyone is looking at, and judging, them.

3. The pressure of college, whether self-imposed, or parental, can cause feelings of inadequacy. Striving to achieve the "perfect" diet and body can create a sense of accomplishment for certain individuals. Food can also be used as a form of self-punishment for not feeling "good enough" or "worthy" of care.

4. Though it is not true of everyone, another reason for ED development is the aversion (whether or not it is conscious) to growing up and dealing with normal adult things like bills, laundry, and scheduling appointments. The ED is a way to revert back to needing to be cared for like a child (or experiencing the childhood the person never really had).

What is the hardest thing about recovery?

"Overcoming the feeling of isolation by finding an ever-supportive and encouraging community that will lift you up. I got to a point where I felt so hopeless that I didn't want to wake up another day because dealing with any type of food was exhausting. In moments like that, it is hard to see the light at the end of the tunnel—but you need to decide within yourself that recovery is worth pursuing and you owe it to yourself to give it a true, honest effort. The moment I realized I needed help was the moment I could see the light at the end of the tunnel, and recovery finally seemed possible."

—A student in recovery from bulimia nervosa

What an eating disorder looks like

What are some things you want to watch out for as you (or loved ones) go off to school?

- You skip meals regularly
- You think about food more than two hours a day, or constantly think about previous and future meals
- You start calorie counting or being obsessed with other means of quantifying food (like macros or food weights/ measures)
- You can't take days off your exercise plan even if sick, tired, or fun plans with friends come up
- You use feeling full of food as a way to numb-out/not feel emotions
- You use feeling hungry as a way to numb-out/not feel emotions
- Your choices of what you allow yourself to eat have become fewer and fewer
- You have to compensate for eating by "getting rid of" what you ate
- Your coffee/tea/diet soda/gum consumption has drastically increased as your caloric intake decreases
- You avoid eating with others because you feel anxious or judged by others about what you eat
- You eat the same foods every day, or have a limited diet
- You chew and spit out food without swallowing to "save calories"
- You switched to a vegetarian or vegan diet to have an easier time turning down food (or have chosen another strict diet plan)
- You feel out of control around food, and perhaps try to avoid it

- You feel guilt or shame for eating
- You create new rituals around food like cutting it into tiny pieces or only eating off certain dishes or with specific utensils

While this is not an exhaustive list, any of these behaviors would be a red flag. I'd want to talk to you and see what is going on.

EDD: Eating Disorder Denial

Thinking this is not you? That you don't really have a problem? Well, I certainly hope so, but look again.

Throughout my career, I have seen a ton of clients who "look" fine on the outside, but actually need psychological and often medical care. This got me thinking about the lies that the eating disorder voice tells us. Like many others, I call this voice "Ed" for short. Ed wants to be in control and will tell you lies to keep up the disease process.

Have you ever heard the voice in your head say:

"You're not thin enough yet."

"You are not sick enough/you're not as sick as [that other person]."

"Your heart rate is so low because you work out so much."

"You're doing fine, you can [insert disordered behavior] more [often/more strictly]."

"You haven't ended up in the hospital yet, you're good."

"You're the exception to the complications, it won't happen to you."

Or something similar?

These are often precursors to the downfall of health.

Recently, I saw an athlete dealing with bulimia who had such low levels of iron in her blood that she needed an immediate blood transfusion in the emergency room. (Thank you to the amazing doctor I work with for catching it.) I had another client peeing reddish urine with a "puffy" body that was hot to the touch. We believe she was doing damage to her kidneys from restricting. Another was having severe gastrointestinal issues that are most likely due to years of laxative abuse and restricting. It was misdiagnosed as gastroparesis until she finally saw a specialist.

What did all of these clients have in common? They said they were "fine" and didn't need to go to the doctor. They weren't "that sick."

This is what scares me. How many people are walking around with serious medical issues that they have found a way to normalize?

If you relate to anything I just said, you are in the right place.

> ★ **Don't wait to seek help. You have to be your own health advocate!**
>
> PSA: Tell all of your providers, from primary care physician, to specialists, therapists, and dietitians about your eating disorder. Yes, even if you haven't told anyone else. We can't help you if we don't know what is going on, and some providers won't ask. I created a handy form you can use to start the conversation with your professionals if you are not sure where to start or are afraid to bring up your eating or other self-harming behaviors.

Eating disorders are diagnosed based on criteria in the *Diagnostic and Statistical Manual of Mental Disorders* (as of 2019, we are on the 5th edition), but you don't need a formal diagnosis to be struggling with your relationship to food or your body.

You might be thinking, "Yeah, but I'm different. This [behavior] works for me."

Oh, honey.

Denial is totally normal when engaged in an eating disorder. This happens when the brain starts becoming malnourished. Research by Dr. Ovidio Bermudez shows us that when we restrict our food intake, our brain actually starts to shrink! This shrinkage starts happening within weeks of not meeting our caloric needs and changes how we think, making our thoughts more rigid (including our food behaviors), and creating a sense of "I'm the exception to the rule." Even the most logical scientific evidence can be twisted to fit the agenda of the ED.

This makes it much harder for the person to admit they even have a problem, let alone want to actually get help for it. Have you noticed that it is harder to concentrate on tasks? That your food rules are increasing? That you are irritable with people? We're not meant to exert so much control and willpower over food. The good news is this is almost entirely reversible with good nutrition and a dose of self-awareness.

What are you avoiding?

Disordered eating and eating disorders are not really about food. EDs are a behavioral way to cope with something else going on in your life, including difficult emotions and feelings. Take some time to think about what your ED is doing for you, both in a positive and negative way. Food behaviors and body image obsession are both symptoms of something else that you are not fully prepared to handle. What is the purpose of your ED? What is it protecting you from? How is it helping you? When you can figure out what reward you're getting from your ED, you can look for healthier ways to get that "reward."

Oftentimes, eating disorders are a way to cope with not having to deal with emotions, whether this is from past trauma or a current emotional state. These are different reasons that people use different behaviors to cope.

Drunkorexia

While it's not its own diagnosis, "drunkorexia" is a term coined for people who "save" their calories for alcohol (instead of food).

Because alcohol contains calories, there has been a trend, primarily among college students, to eat lightly (or in some cases, skipping food altogether!) on days they know they are going to be drinking a lot, in attempt to avoid weight gain, or to heighten the effect of alcohol.

Don't fall into this dangerous trap! Not only does alcohol not provide necessary nutrients for sustaining life, it can be deadly!

Please, please, eat before or while you're drinking, drink water, and try not to binge drink. It may seem "fun" or like "everyone is doing it," but you can be a good example for everyone else (and you will thank yourself in the morning!).

The binge-restrict cycle (it's a trap!)

A theme that comes up often in my practice is the "binge-restrict cycle." I literally have it drawn on the back of every notepad I own. Illustrated below, this cycle is the same for most people with food issues. The behaviors vary, but the concept remains the same.

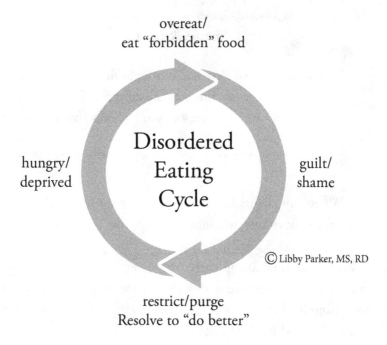

overeat/
eat "forbidden" food

hungry/
deprived

Disordered
Eating
Cycle

guilt/
shame

© Libby Parker, MS, RD

restrict/purge
Resolve to "do better"

It starts with restricting, dieting, or "being good" (bottom of circle) by limiting what you eat, eating "clean," compensating for eating, or other means of creating rules for yourself with food. This leads to feeling physically hungry (the body still has to eat, even if you are trying to override that need) or deprived. The result is overeating, binge eating, or eating "forbidden" foods that we told ourselves we can't have (for whatever arbitrary reason). In fact, Dr. Neumark-Sztainer, author of *I'm, Like, So Fat!*, remarked that frequent dieting among teen girls creates a 12-fold increase in the likelihood of binge eating as opposed to girls who don't diet. Binge eating (or eating "forbidden foods") creates feelings of shame and guilt. This drives the compulsion to make up for it and "do better" so that it doesn't happen again.

And round and round we go.

Shame & Guilt

Do you know the difference? I thought they were basically the same until recently, but they are different. Shame means you think YOU are a bad person. Guilt means you think your ACTIONS were bad.

When my clients have tried to interrupt this cycle on their own, they inevitably attempt to stop the binge or eating of the "bad" food. Usually, by the time they get to me, they are so exhausted from using their willpower to try to stop binging that they can't even see a different route to fixing things. The overeating is what is causing the distress, right? It causes the guilt, shame, and self-loathing, right?

Wrong! The cause of the whole cycle is the restriction piece. Whether it is the true definition of restriction (not consuming enough calories or nutrients to thrive) or depriving yourself of the foods you like (cutting out specific foods or food groups, including dieting) or even compensation for eating by vomiting or over-exercising, this "restriction" creates mental deprivation and physical hunger. The funny thing is that most people fall into this cycle as a result of wanting to regulate or lose weight when, invariably, the restrictions lead to rebound weight gain—the exact opposite of the intention.

It is well documented that losing weight beyond what our body naturally wants to do (our body's "set point") is difficult if not impossible to maintain, and inevitably leads to rebound weight gain of equal or greater amounts, as the body starts preparing for what it perceives as famine. The fact is our body doesn't know if we are in a true famine or on a diet.

To stop the cycle, we must stop the restriction phase. If you are eating enough and not depriving yourself, you won't feel that gnawing hunger and won't overdo it; and if you don't overdo it, you won't feel the shame or guilt and won't need to restrict!

I know it is easier said than done, but stick with me. If you commit, you can get out of this cycle and shake ED for good. It's a long process, but well worth it.

It all starts with learning to listen to your body.

What is the hardest thing about recovery?

"Learning to enjoy food again. Really enjoy it. The cooking, the smells, the cravings, all of it. It's so sad when you want to enjoy what you are eating, but your brain is screaming terrible things at you. My heart wanted to love food, and my brain wouldn't let me."

—Young woman recovering from anorexia

Main takeaways:

- Eating disorders are a way to cope with something the person wants to avoid or control.
- It's common for people suffering from an eating disorder to think they don't have a problem.
- Our body doesn't know the difference between famine and a diet and will try to keep weight on when deprived.
- To stop overeating or binging, you have to stop depriving yourself.

Take action (grab your journal):

Journal about what your ED is doing for you in both a positive and negative way. What is the purpose of your ED? What is it protecting you from? How is it helping you?

Notice what food beliefs you have. What do you allow or not allow yourself to have? What rules have you given yourself around food (such as timing or calories)? Write them down.

Does eating or eating certain foods cause you shame or guilt?

Did any of the signs of disordered eating (that list) stand out for you? If so, which ones? Any that I didn't mention?

Chapter 2

Are You Listening?

"The hardest step she ever took was to blindly trust in who she was."

—Atticus

If I could grant you one realistic wish, I wish that you would trust your body. Since the beginning of human existence, we've had to trust our body's own biofeedback mechanisms to tell us things like when to sleep, drink, eat, how much to eat, and when to stop. However, somewhere along the way you, like most people, lost faith in your magnificent body.

I'm guessing you have a good grasp on what *really hungry* and *really stuffed* feel like. You know what putting on the stretchy pants feels like, and when you're so hungry you might (or do!) faint.

But what about the in-between?

Hunger and fullness are a spectrum, not two finite settings. We can be a little peckish, content, comfortably full, and experience many other states of hunger and fullness.

You might be saying, "But I don't feel those levels! I only feel [stuffed/ravenous]." Never fear! You can again. We are all born with the innate ability to determine when we are still hungry and when we are getting full. And while we might forget it over time, it's possible to relearn.

So how do we figure out our hunger and fullness cues? Every individual has slightly different ways that they notice hunger and fullness in their body. For some people, feeling hungry could be a lightheadedness or inability to concentrate. It could be lethargy, tiredness, stomach grumbling, or stomach pangs.

Fullness may also leave you feeling tired. Your stomach may hurt from pressure, you may no longer want to think of food, your breathing may change, or you may just feel content. Fullness, like hunger, can look like a lot of different things, but what's important is that you start tuning into *your* body and noticing what hunger and fullness feel like to *you*.

There's a wide range of hunger and fullness. It is not an on-off switch where we're either hungry or we are full. So, if you're using the food and feelings journal that's included with this book (more on that later in the chapter), there's a place for your degree of hunger before and after each meal. This is noted on a scale of 1 to 10, with 1 being so starving you would eat anything put in front of you, 10 being so full you're unbuttoning your pants, and 5 is pretty neutral. If you are recovering from disordered eating, don't expect to get this right away. And if you have been under eating, you will need to push past fullness for the time being. More on that in a little bit.

Notice how you feel before and after you eat. It can take a while to get back to trusting your body, but we're all born with the ability to know when we're hungry and when we're full. If you think of a baby, they will cry when they're hungry and want food. When they're full, you can't push any more food into them. They will pull away from it.

We all have the ability to get back to that state. The fact that we struggle to feel our hunger is typically related to social constraints, as we are told many times of the day whether it's appropriate to eat or not. This can screw up our hunger and fullness cues if we let them get out of hand. Each time we eat, we can ask, "Am I hungry? How hungry am I? Do I just need a little bit of food? Do I need a full meal?"

Additionally, think about how hungry you are as you eat a meal. Typically, somewhere in the meal, we have a point where we naturally pause and take a breath. For most of us, that's a good stopping point. That's when we're feeling pretty full. Satiety takes some time to notice, so try waiting for 15 to 20 minutes to see if you are still hungry before reaching for seconds. Sometimes, we will push through and continue to eat because that's where we're at that day, and that's okay, too.

Something interesting to note is that we have different mechanisms in place in our gastrointestinal system, our gustatory system (how our gut senses food), and our olfactory system (smell perception) to feel hunger and fullness. For example, after you've had a couple of bites of a certain food, you'll be less hungry for it. This is good because it encourages us to eat a variety of different foods. As you'll notice, food will start to taste less good as you continue to eat it. The first bite of cake is always better than the 20th bite of cake. So, if you can enjoy the first couple of bites, that will help you stop before you get over-full. What I'm describing here is considered mindful eating.

Recognizing hunger and fullness cues can be difficult if you haven't been doing it for a while, especially if you have been restricting what you eat for a long time. I recommend writing down what physical sensations you feel as you notice them, so you can start seeing patterns. But first, some more about how our body processes food.

Hunger: physical need to eat

Appetite: psychological desire to eat (or not: "lack of appetite")

Satiety: feeling of fullness and satisfaction

The stretchy stomach

It's important to understand the physiology of our body to understand hunger and fullness.

Our stomach is made of elaborately folded muscle that stretches and holds anywhere from about a tablespoon of food and fluid up to a liter in capacity. That's quite a range! When we put food and fluid into our stomach, the stretch receptors in the cells making up the lining of the stomach send a signal up to the brain, which the brain reads as, "We're getting full, stop eating."

But how can we recognize real fullness? And why do some people register fullness very quickly while others tackle huge eating contests without ever feeling full? What's going on?

Physiologically, our stomach has adapted to a "normal" amount (volume) of food that we typically eat (our typical meal size). If we're eating average portions of food, our stomach is going to sit somewhere in the middle of this range, and when we eat enough food to fill the volume of the stomach, the stomach walls will stretch. This signals the feeling of "I'm full," and our brain tells us to stop eating.

For people who chronically overeat, the stomach has been stretched more than others. Therefore, it takes more food and fluids to push the sides of the stomach and trigger those stretch receptors to signal the brain to stop eating. Because of this, we can eat enough to be adequately nourished but still not feel totally full.

On the flip side, for people who have no appetite or are restricting their intake, their stomach may have become smaller. This will make it more difficult to eat enough to be nourished, as they will feel full after consuming a very small amount food and fluid.

The good news is that stomach volume is totally changeable. Our stomach capacity will change throughout our lives. For instance, if we're under-eating and our stomach has shrunk, we can train ourselves to eat larger and larger portions, pushing past fullness a little bit each time. But what about when you honestly feel full soon after you start eating? Stuffing yourself can work, but you may feel sick and find that it's too much to handle, especially if the eating disorder voice is strong. You can work around this uncomfortable experience by adding as little as two bites to each eating occasion (past fullness), which will start to stretch the stomach back out towards "normal."

I call this my *"2-Bite Rule."*

Why two bites? It is enough to slowly add up (if you do it every time you eat), without being too uncomfortable. It will slowly stretch the stomach back to a normal size, making eating easier and more comfortable.

What you need to do:

- When we need to eat more, but the stomach says "FULL!" gently push yourself by eating two more bites than you feel you have space for.
- Do this at each meal and snack, until you work up to eating the full portion sizes/meal plan your dietitian has

recommended (or you get to adequate portion sizes—be honest!—if not working with an RD yet).

- These two extra bites are not too much to cause pain, but are slowly stretching your stomach back out so that you can gradually work up to eating full meals again. (If you want to be an overachiever, try for three more bites.)

Several clients that I have worked with have had great success using this tactic to get their stomach back on track.

*Disclaimer: If you are in a treatment program or working with a dietitian, please follow the instructions or meal plan set specifically for you. This is not for everyone.

If, on the other hand, you're eating too much right now or you're binging, it might take a lot to feel full (if you signal fullness at all). When that happens, you may need to stop eating a bit before you get to the point of fullness and bring your stomach back down. If you suddenly cut back on food, you're going to be absolutely starving, so you need to train your body very slowly. In this case, we can reverse the 2-Bite Rule, and eat two fewer bites than normal at each eating occasion.

Hara Hachi Bu

If you struggle with habitual overeating, try the Japanese practice of *hara hachi bu*, which means eating until you are 80 percent full. Add another layer of mindfulness; what does 80 percent, or even 85 percent full feel like? How do you tell yourself to stop?

Some tips to assist you:

- Before doing it, see what's eating you. Are you eating for comfort? Numbing yourself? *Hara hachi bu* won't fix those things. (Find out more about dealing with this in chapter 7.)
- Eat slowly. When we eat rapidly, we cannot register fullness as fast as we eat. This almost always leads to feeling overfull a half-hour later. Try setting your fork down between bites. Engage in conversation while you eat.
- Don't eat right out of the package. Portion out how much food you think you will eat on a plate or bowl and put the package away. (Important note: It does not have to be the serving size on the package! It is okay if it's more than the listed "portion size." These are manufacturing reference numbers, not necessarily consumption portions.)
- Try eating mindfully. Focus on the food and limit distractions. What is the taste? Texture? Smell? How did the ingredients grow? (I have a guided mindfulness exercise to help you in chapter 5.)

G.I. issues

During long-term restriction, a lot of people feel like they have (or even get diagnosed with) IBS (irritable bowel syndrome). Symptoms include gas, constipation or diarrhea, bloating, and sometimes stomachaches. Funny thing is, it typically resolves after eating normalizes.

Whether or not these issues came up during restrictive phases of eating or after a period of restriction, there are some gastrointestinal (G.I.) issues that many people notice. Luckily, these tend to be short lived, as long as you keep eating and don't fall back into restriction.

Typical things you may experience when eating more after a phase of restriction:

- **Bloating or gas:** There are many potential causes, such as water retention and/or slowed digestion while your gut relearns how to handle food or fast additions of fiber-rich fruits and veggies. Also, when restricting, your gut microbiota (the good bacteria in your gut) are reduced. Since they are an essential part of digestion, more gas may be produced during the digestion process.
- **Early feeling of fullness:** Your stomach is totally capable of eating large volumes of food, but it needs to stretch back out. Stretch receptors in the stomach signal the brain that it is "full," even if not truly full and nourished.
- **Nausea or unintended regurgitation:** Especially if you have made yourself throw up before, or after eating quickly (side effects of physical or psychological restriction).

- **Constipation:** Especially if you have abused laxatives—your colon starts depending on laxatives to poop at all!
- **Diarrhea:** Often occurs from changes in gut microbiota, or excessive amounts of "sugar-free" foods, which contain sugar alcohols. Sugar alcohols are not fully absorbed in the G.I. tract and ferment, which creates a laxative-like effect (along with gas or bloating).
- **Slow gastric transit time:** The stomach empties slowly into the small intestine, creating a longer feeling of fullness, and often constipation.
- **Heartburn/acid reflux:** Until the stomach is comfortably stretched back to normal, the low volume capacity can cause some acid to splash up from the stomach when eating more than you have been. This is also a common side effect for those who vomit a lot and can cause long-term damage to the esophagus and teeth. The cessation of purging will slowly reduce acid reflux. Anxiety is another trigger for reflux.
- **Hypermetabolism:** Sped-up metabolic rate, which may cause excessive sweating especially at night, or a feeling that you are "burning" everything you eat quickly. This tends to subside back to a "normal" metabolism after eating enough for a year or more.
- **Edema:** "Puffiness" caused by fluid in the tissue, typically around the face and ankles. This is caused by issues related to the fluid balance between cells, and often results from a protein imbalance.
- **Swollen cheeks:** "Puffy face" or "chipmunk cheeks," if you were vomiting. The parotid glands in the cheeks and throat swell with regular vomiting. This goes away a week or so after not vomiting.

- **Increased anxiety:** Eating more. 'Nuff said. This gets better—keep eating!

The G.I. tract issues are typically caused by lack of use. Our G.I. tract is essentially a long tube of muscles which, like other muscles, falls into the "use it or lose it" category. When you don't eat certain foods, don't eat as much food, or don't have full strength due to malnutrition, your G.I. tract needs to rebuild strength from proper nutrition and regular use.

The good news is these issues do go away over time if you continue to eat enough and don't restrict. What I often see is that one or more of these complications occurs and the person gets so scared that they go back to restricting, which only prolongs the issue. The more you go back to restricting, the longer these issues will last.

What is the hardest thing about recovery?

"Trying to pretend to the outside world that I'm fine [when] I'm living a double life; having a constant series of calculations going on in my head and making myself eat when it's the last thing I want to do."

—Anonymous

Something that happens for many people early in recovery, especially those who have been restricting what they eat, is a quasi "binge" period. This can look like days of feeling like you can't get full, no matter how much you eat, followed by days of being afraid you are eating too much and trying to restrict again.

Like a pendulum, it can swing back and forth while your body figures out what feels good. This doesn't mean that you are, or will, develop a binge eating disorder. Often, we just need to let it shake out before we land in the middle where food peace exists.

Intuitive eating

The ultimate goal is getting back to a place of intuitive eating. As previously stated, we are all born knowing when we are hungry or full and what we need—then life messes it up. Intuitive eating, simply put, is listening to, and trusting, your body to tell you what it needs. There are whole books and courses on the "principles of intuitive eating," (and I encourage you to read them) but to sum it up, all you really need is trust.

If you are listening to your body, you won't need to binge or restrict. It won't ask you for candy all the time. If you listen, your body will sometimes ask for candy (or whatever), but it will also ask for vegetables and proteins. It will ask for rest and for activity. When you can be in harmony with your body, you will be happier than you ever were on any diet.

You have permission to eat. I know you might feel afraid of certain foods, but all foods fit in a healthy lifestyle and provide nutrition. I mean it.

Now that you have an idea of how to listen to your body (and don't worry about mastering this yet—this can take a while), let's move on to meal planning, but not the way you might think.

How it feels to have a healthy relationship with food

"It has been quite some time since I had a healthy relationship with food. There has always been a battle in my mind—"Eat this not that. You're not hungry, you're just bored. You need to stay in caloric deficit"—until I was referred to Libby and she slowly introduced me to what I know now as intuitive eating. Now, instead of being fearful of my body's signs of hunger, I have come to recognize those signs as opportunities to fuel my body appropriately, which differs day to day. Not being scared of my appetite or food in general has helped curb those insatiable cravings and has given me balance in eating and other areas of life. Knowing and trusting your body is so freeing."

—Kate Scott

Food & Feelings Journal

What we do want to focus on, rather than numbers, is having generally balanced meals and days. To do that, we can use a powerful tool: the food and feelings journal.

Food Journal for: Today's Date:

© Not Your Average Nutitionist, LLC

Time/ Where/ Who is Present	Degree of Hunger Before*	Before Thoughts/ Feelings/ Etc.	Food/ Beverage Eaten	Degree of Hunger After*	After Thoughts/ Feelings/ Etc.

*Scale 1-10, 1=Starving, 10=Stuffed

★ The food and feelings journal is something that you can use alone or with a dietitian or a therapist to help you with your relationship with food. While anyone can use it, I have designed it specifically for people with disordered eating. The journal is designed to help you to look objectively at what you are eating as well as related patterns. These include your triggers, thoughts, and feelings about food as well as hunger and fullness levels. So, let's dive in and see what we need to put into these different spots.

You can download a PDF version of the journal or make your own in your journal or on the computer.

On the left side of your paper, write down what time (approximately) you've starting eating, if you're with anyone or if you're alone, and where you are eating. Are you alone in your room? Are you at the kitchen table? Whether in a restaurant, in a cafeteria, at a friend's house, or outside, go ahead and put that in the box. Where we are and who we are with can change how we eat. Make comparisons with other locations and people or scenarios to see the influence it has on your eating habits.

The next column is degree of hunger or fullness before eating. This is ranked on a scale of 1 to 10, with 1 being absolutely starving, you're ready to gnaw your arm off, and 10 being so stuffed you couldn't eat another bite and are considering unbuttoning your pants. 5 is neutral—at 5, you could eat a little more, but you don't need to, you're really content. Go back and review the hunger and fullness cues section as needed.

Ideally after, or in between meals, we're feeling a range between 4 and 7. That's a really nice, comfortable space. If you're getting below 3 or 4, you'll want to be eating pretty soon, and if you're above a 7 or 8, you'll want to stop eating (or we're a little full and that's okay for now).

It can be really hard to know your degree of hunger and fullness. Don't beat yourself up if it's difficult. The more you practice this, the easier it will be to tell if you're hungry or full. Just the simple fact of checking in with yourself is important. Most of us don't check in with ourselves, but the more we do it, the easier it becomes.

Our next column is thoughts, feelings, and emotions before eating. This does not have to be related to food, but it can be. List what you are feeling as you're preparing your food or getting ready to eat. Is there any anxiety around it? Are you thinking you're not eating what you "should" be eating (a little hint here: try not to "should" yourself)? Also, consider if you're feeling really excited. Did a happy situation occur? Are you celebrating? Are you angry because you just found out that your parents are getting a divorce? Emotions like these could strongly affect your intake.

The next column is food and beverage eaten. This is very loosely structured. I don't want this to be a calorie or macro counting thing for you. In fact, please, DON'T list numbers on here. The way you write down your food and beverage can vary depending on what you're comfortable with and your purpose. If you're just using this for yourself, you can write it down however you want. If you're using it with a dietitian, it's a good idea to have some portion reference written down. For example, if you're just using it for yourself, you could write down a turkey sandwich, but if you're working with a dietitian, you'll want to write out "two slices of [specific brand] bread, five slices of deli turkey, a tablespoon of mayo, some lettuce and tomato."

Make sure to list any beverages that have calories in them, by which I mean anything that's not water. Hopefully, you are drinking water. If so, logging it can be optional. If you struggle with drinking enough water, this may be a useful thing to include. Alternatively, if you overhydrate or "fluid load" it is also helpful to note.

Hydration

As a general rule, the standard eight 8 oz glasses of water per day is a good place to start. More may be needed if you sweat a lot, are in a really hot environment, or are eating a lot more than the average person. Pretty much all fluids (except alcohol) count toward our hydration needs. Water, tea, coffee, milk, fruits and veggies with high water content, broth-based soup, juice, hot chocolate, sports beverages all count towards your hydration needs.

Dehydration

Even two percent dehydration can lead to brain fog, lethargy, and suboptimal body function. Yet, many restrictive eaters also restrict fluids in attempt to lower body weight or punish themselves. First of all, water weight is not fat, so losing water is just that—losing water. Water is required for cleaving apart food molecules in the process of digestion. If you are chronically dehydrated, you run the risk of fainting or shutting down body functions (to the point of death). We NEED water!

Overhydration

Overhydrating, or fluid-loading, is a dangerous behavior. Whether on purpose or not, having too much fluid in your system thins out blood and can lead to water intoxication and death!

When hydrating, especially when exercising over an hour or sweating a lot, make sure to have electrolytes along with your water. Sports beverages help (not the zero-calorie options!). They include carbohydrate (six to eight percent is optimal), sodium, potassium, and usually some other electrolytes to help maintain blood electrolyte levels.

Caffeine

Caffeine is an overused substance among those with EDs. The 2015 recommendations for dietary guidelines state that up to approximately 400 mg of caffeine per day (three to five cups of drip coffee) for HEALTHY adults (up to 85 mg for children and adolescents) is fine to consume. However, if you are not eating enough, have heart issues, or are on certain medications, caffeine needs to be limited. Energy drinks are not advised for anyone, healthy or not. Other ingredients in energy drinks have a compounding effect with caffeine, which can send the consumer into cardiac arrest!

Next, after the column on what food we ate, we have another evaluation of our degree of hunger or fullness. You can note this immediately after eating, or up to half an hour after. You want to see how full that food made you feel in relation to the degree of hunger before you ate and then record thoughts and feelings. It is particularly interesting to me, as a dietitian, to see what's coming up afterwards, especially over time. For example, do you have less anxiety and guilt about what you ate over the weeks? Or is it getting worse? Are we seeing certain patterns emerge, for example, around thoughts you had before eating or people you're eating with?

The whole purpose of using the food and feelings journal is to look objectively at all of this data over time. Therefore, we don't want to take any one occasion as a big deal. Once you have several days' or weeks' worth of journal entries, review the data you've collected. Notice I did not say "guilt collected."

Some data to observe:

You may notice you eat alone a lot as a way to avoid social eating situations. Why is that? What are you missing out on?

Maybe you eat lightly all day long and stuff yourself to feelings of guilt most nights. What would happen if you ate earlier in the day? (Hint: your night gorge will likely decrease!)

When you are stressed or anxious, do you eat your feelings or do you get really picky about food and hardly eat? Food is not going to change the situation. What can you do instead that will actually help your specific situation? (More on this in chapter 7.)

In the next chapter, we will go into the specifics of creating balanced meals with foods you actually like (not just the ones you tell yourself you like because they are "healthy").

Main takeaways:

- How your body tells you it is hungry and full, and what this looks like on a spectrum.
- G.I. issues usually resolve as you return to normal eating.

- Your feelings and situations affect how you eat.

Take action (grab your journal):

Print out or write in your food and feelings journal. Keep a log of at least three days (a week or two is better) if it is not triggering. Only after several days do I want you to go back and look at what you wrote.

For this week, I want you to focus on how hungry you are, particularly before eating. Try to log it. Work up to how hungry you feel before AND after eating.

Did you fully satisfy your hunger? Were you hungry for food or for something else? Do you need to eat a little bit more? And before the meal, how hungry are you? Do you need a little bit of food? Do you need a full meal? Do you not want anything at all, but you're eating because it's time to eat?

Start paying attention to the cues, even if you're not taking action on them right now. The more aware you are of your body and your personal needs, the more you can move toward making changes.

Have you noticed any G.I. issues? After reading this chapter, do you have a better idea of why they might be occurring?

Chapter 3

Meal Planning Without Planning

"One cannot think well, love well, sleep well, if one has not dined well."

—Virginia Woolf

H ey, you.

Yes you, sitting there thinking about what to eat. I have a message for you—there are no bad foods.

Let me repeat that: *There. Are. No. Bad. Foods.*

Food has no moral value. Are some foods more nutritious than others? Absolutely, I'm not denying that; but our body will take nutrients out of every food. The term "empty calories" doesn't make sense. Calories are units of energy, they are not "empty" but rather a variation on carbohydrates, proteins, and fats. Do we need some foods in greater proportion to others for optimal health? Yes, but all foods are part of a healthy diet.[1]

This can be a real mindset shift for some people who have dieted or been told there are "good" and "bad" foods. Foods do not have moral value, they cannot be good or bad. This just accentuates black-or-white thinking, a common cognitive distortion. If it is safe (not causing foodborne illness, or allergy), it is not going to hurt you to eat it.

I think the reason many people have "fear foods" or believe in "good" versus "bad" foods is that they overeat or binge on the so-called bad foods and find it is easier to avoid them altogether. This is the foundation for disordered eating. When we deprive ourselves or say we can't have something, it sets us up to want it more. If we deprive ourselves of the specific food, or enough food, we almost inevitably overeat when our willpower runs out (which is typically at the end of the day, this being the reason why most people binge or "cheat on their diet" at night). Go back and look at the binge-restrict cycle in chapter 1.

We cannot rely on willpower, and honestly if it takes that much work to stay on a specific eating plan, it's not going to be sustainable and you are going to be miserable trying to keep it up. If you incorporate all kinds of foods into your daily diet, you are far less likely to crave them or overeat.

1 My two exceptions to "all foods are fit": 1) Trans fats. Avoid them, as our body cannot process them; but trace amounts won't hurt you, and they will be out of all foods by 2020. 2) Energy drinks. They can cause arrhythmias and death because of the compounding effect of the herbal ingredients in the caffeine, which send thousands of people into cardiac arrest every year.

Incorporating "fear foods"

If it is overwhelming to think of incorporating a fear food because you are afraid of overeating, especially sweets, try this proven method: Have a portion of the food (for example, one cookie or a few small pieces of candy) right before lunch. Finish your meal with something savory (like vegetables or meat), so the sweet taste is not still in your mouth. This will ensure you're less likely to overeat the fear food. By having a fear food on a daily basis, you are taking away its power over you. Over time, it becomes just another food. Eventually, you can have it whenever you want just because it sounds good, not because you are compelled to binge on it.

If we strip away the labels we put on food and make it just one part of our life among others, we will be less stressed, healthier, and at a natural weight for our unique body.

A different way of looking at meals—through a dancer's eyes

Whether you are a dancer in the formal sense or you bust a move at a party (or your bedroom), you probably move your body. So let me ask you this:

Would you do the exact same one or two moves over and over for a whole song?

If you have a dancer's eye, the answer is clearly, NO!

Why?

A few reasons: You would get bored and the people watching would get bored. What's more, doing the same repetitive movement without balancing it out would increase your risk of injury.

So why do you eat the same foods every day? It's the same thing, but it impacts you more than a pulled muscle. The body is designed to eat a variety of foods the same way it is designed to move in a variety of ways. Many people with eating disorders end up eating the same set of limited foods every day because it is "safe."

But we don't grow if we don't change it up.

Like a dance that has dynamics, drama, and a series of varying moves, our meals should encompass a variety of foods that also change from day to day. So just like you wouldn't do an entire song of barrel turns, your whole week shouldn't consist of eating the same few foods.

Start expanding your comfort zone, branch out into new foods that will nourish your body. Try picking a variety of foods at each meal. Choose different food groups, colors, textures, and see if you find some new dishes you love.

See what combinations of food you can "choreograph" at your meals.

★ Meal planning without "planning"

I'm going to teach you an easy way to meal plan on the fly. This meal plan, called the "Rule of 3s," was developed by Marcia Herrin and Maria Larkin in the book, *Nutrition Counseling in the Treatment of Eating Disorders,* a bible for dietitians working in the eating disorders field. Based on their extensive experience, they developed a plan that works for most people. I love this plan because it gives structure to create balanced meals without telling you exactly what to eat. Obviously, no meal plan fits everyone, but for the majority of people, this fits really well because there are no specific portion sizes tied to it. Based on their research, I developed a worksheet that I'll share with you here.

Rule of 3s Meal Plan

Adapted from: Herrin & Larkin, *Nutrition Counseling in the Treatment of Eating Disorders*

BREAKFAST		
Calcium		
Grain or Starch		
Fruit or Vegetable		
Protein (opt.)		
Fat (opt.)		
SNACK		
LUNCH		
Calcium		
Grain or Starch		
Fruit or Vegetable		
Protein		
Fat		
Fun Food		

SNACK		
DINNER		
Calcium		
Grain or Starch		
Fruit or Vegetable		
Protein		
Fat		
Fun Food		
SNACK		

worksheet by: Not Your Average Nutitionist, LLC

We're going to look at our different categories of food groups or nutrients as they're broken down into three meals and three snacks. If you're hitting all of the food groups in these different sections, you'll be pretty balanced and well nourished. This worksheet is going to give you the space to come up with two days of example meals, broken down into different categories. So very briefly, let's walk through the different categories to ensure you know what you're looking for.

Our first category is calcium. Calcium is a super important mineral to consume, regardless of whether you eat dairy or not. The reason we want to ensure you're including good sources of calcium at least three times a day is that it facilitates bone growth and development, prevents osteoporosis, and plays an important role in muscle contractions. The very basic need to move and lift things requires calcium. It's an important mineral, and I want to make sure you are getting enough of it.

For most of our lifespan, our calcium needs are roughly 1,000 mg a day; during peak bone-building years (a.k.a. teen years) 1,300 mg a day is necessary. It's important to split this up over the day because we don't want to get all of our calcium at one time. I say this because, like other nutrients, our bodies are not able to fully absorb all the required calcium at once. This applies even if you're taking calcium supplements. Whenever you're dealing with supplements, you'll want to make sure you take them at two different times during the day. For example, if you have 500 mg tablets of calcium (500 to 600 mg is standard), you want to take it twice, one 500 mg tablet in the morning and one 500 mg tablet in the evening. If you're eating dairy or any other calcium source, you will want to have one serving (about one cup of dairy milk or its equivalent) at a time (30 percent DV, or Daily Value, of calcium is an equivalent serving), because that's all your body can really utilize at any one time.

Good sources of calcium

Cow's milk
Cheese
Yogurt
Kefir
Almond Milk
Soy Milk
Calcium-fortified orange juice

*Look for at least 30 percent of your DV per serving on the nutrition facts label.
**Vitamin D helps with calcium absorption. Many food products have vitamin D added for this reason.
***All supplements are not created equal. Ideally, you get your vitamins from real food. If you do need a calcium supplement, a combination of calcium citrate plus vitamin D is best absorbed by the body.

Our next category is grains or starch. I know a lot of you are probably afraid of these foods because they're villainized in the media, but they're very, very important.[2] Grains and starches have carbohydrate molecules and a lot of essential B vitamins that we need for bodily processes, including brain function. B vitamins are actually essential to metabolism (breaking down food into energy). B vitamins are also necessary for making and repairing DNA and RNA, synthesizing neurochemicals and signal molecules in the body and brain, developing the nervous system, and more.

If we need to be using our brain for school, our job, or life in general, we need to have the glucose from carbohydrates in our bloodstream for processing and faster reaction time. In fact, having low calories or carbs can actually make it harder to think logically! Grains and starches are a really easy way to ensure these needs are met. Additionally, carbohydrates give us the energy needed to move and to exercise. So, we want to be sure we're getting carbohydrates in each meal and snack.

Better choices for grains and starches are ones that are used in their whole form because whole grains contain fiber. Fiber helps us feel full, keeps our bowel movements regular by bulking our feces, and is wonderful for colon health, including the fact that it helps to prevent colon cancer. I like to think of fiber as a Brillo pad for scrubbing the colon clean.

---

2 It seems like each decade has a different "food villain." In the 2010s it is carbohydrates, especially from sugar. The '80s and '90s it was fats, and even things like solid foods ('80s), or other crazy food fads—remember the "cabbage soup diet"? Yuck! Are proteins the next "villain" as we overdo it on protein foods with the current fads?

Examples of grains and starches

Rice
Bread
Tortillas
Beans and legumes (like lentils)
Potatoes
Peas
Corn
Quinoa
Pastries
Oatmeal
Crackers
Cold cereals
Squash

*For more whole grains, check out
https://wholegrainscouncil.org/.
**Ideally, most of your choices are 100 percent whole grain,
but there is plenty of space for non–whole grain foods in a
healthy diet.

The next category is fruits and vegetables. I'm not going to go into too much depth here. We've all been told our entire life that we need to eat our fruits and veggies, and there are a lot of reasons for it. I do want to note that we want to be eating the rainbow of colors in fruits and vegetables. Don't ignore the different colors. Each color has a different purpose with different compounds that make them very healthy for us. So, try to eat as much of a variety of produce as you can. Get all the different colors—red, orange, yellow, green, blue, purple, white. See what new types of fruits and vegetables you can incorporate into your diet. Mix it up.

A small sampling of fruits and vegetables

Tomatoes
Oranges
Bell peppers
Salad greens (all kinds)
Apples
Eggplant
Star fruit
Berries (all kinds)
Cauliflower

*Eat the rainbow, all the different colors have different health benefits. See how many colors you can get in over the course of a week.
**Mushrooms fit in this category for the purpose of this worksheet

---

On to protein. There are many types of protein out there, and different foods have different levels of protein. Proteins (amino acids) are essential for all body processes. They are what makes up our body tissue, including our organs, hair, skin, nails, and muscles. They're also prime components in other bodily functions including hormones, fluid balance between cells, and cofactors for different enzymatic processes in our body.

That being said, most Americans tend to eat too much protein. Protein is just one part of a healthy diet. Only 10 to 35 percent of our calories should come from protein. Like the other nutrients, we can only process and utilize so much protein at once. For most people, up to about 30 grams of protein per meal can be effectively used. Extreme protein intake is unnecessary and will simply lead to more fat accumulation and potentially kidney issues.

Proteins

Meat (1 oz is about 7 g of protein)
Fish
Cheese/milk/yogurt
Eggs (1 large egg is about 7 g of protein)
Tofu/soy
Tempeh
Beans
Nuts/nut butter (2 tbsp of nut butter is about 7 g of protein)
Seeds
Protein powder/bars (in a pinch, but try not to eat as your primary source)

And then we have fats. Dietary fats (fats we eat) are very important. I know they were villainized in the '80s and '90s, but we do need to eat fat in our diet along with foods that have fat-soluble vitamins (A, E, D, and K), which are most often found in vegetables. Fat helps with the absorption of the fat-soluble vitamins. If we don't have fat in our diet, then these vitamins aren't going to be absorbed easily or at all! For example, it's really good to have some fat in your salad. Salad dressing, cheese, avocado, chicken, or another fat source will help with the absorption of fat-soluble vitamins.

With dietary fats, the healthier versions are going to be liquid at room temperature instead of solid. So, our oils, like olive oil or nuts, are a healthier option, and should be selected more frequently than fat that is solid at room temperature, like butter, shortening, or lard (but you can still eat these fats).

Coconut oil is controversial because it lands somewhere in the middle. It has a lower melting point than most of our solid fats, like butter, but it is solid at room temperature because it contains a lot of saturated fatty acids (about 92 percent!). Saturated fats (saturated meaning fully "saturated" with hydrogen atoms instead of having double bonds between carbon atoms) are responsible for the solid structure of fats. Ideally, we should get more unsaturated (fat molecules with double bonds) fats in our diet, which are going to be liquid at room temperature. Coconut oil has a good number of medium-chain triglycerides (MCT), which are more easily absorbed and oxidized by the liver than long-chain triglycerides (LCT). This makes it more desirable than LCTs, and creates the assumption of less fat gain (though this is yet to be proven in a large randomized controlled study).

Dietary fats

Unsaturated (liquid)
Olive oil
Vegetable oil
Avocado
Nuts/nut oils
Seeds (chia, flax, hemp)
Fish oil
Salad dressing

Saturated (solid)
Butter
Coconut oil
Lard
Crisco
Animal fat (marbling in meat, dairy fat)

*Choose unsaturated (liquid at room temperature) oils more often than saturated (solid at room temperature) fats.
**Low-fat dairy is perfectly fine and good for you.

The last category that we have on our sheet is fun food. Fun food can be anything. If there are still a lot of fear foods in your diet, maybe a fun food is a banana. If you're really trying to move on and you're ready to change it up, a fun food could be a brownie, chips, or whatever the heck you want.

Fun foods

Anything goes! What sounds good?

When filling out this worksheet, we have three meals (with subcategories) and three snacks. When we're looking at building a meal, I know it can be overwhelming to see these different categories and think, "OMG. How am I going to meet all of these needs?!" What I have found to be easier is to think of a meal that you already like and break it down into the categories. Did it meet all of the categories or do you still need to add something?

Example: Pizza

Let's break pizza down into these categories. Looking at a traditional slice of pizza, we have calcium as our cheese. Our grain or starch is the pizza crust. Fruits or vegetables may not be on the pizza, so let's skip that for a moment. Do we have protein? Yes, if there's a lot of cheese, or we have some meat or vegetarian protein on there. Great! If there's not very much cheese and no meat or other protein on it, look for another source of protein. And then fat, typically, is the cheese on pizza, especially if there is a lot of cheese or if it's baked with oils.

Our pizza has calcium, grains, and fat. So, we're still looking for fruits, veggies, and maybe some protein. For example, with our slice(s) of pizza, we could add a side salad. That salad will have different vegetables and we can add some protein like slices of a hardboiled egg or chicken. Boom. We have a rounded-out meal. (My favorite kind of pizza, Hawaiian, has pineapple and Canadian bacon, so it hits all the categories.)

Can I be vegan while recovering?

You don't have to cut out any foods that you are not truly allergic to (or for religious reasons—but check yourself on this, too). I have no problems with plant-based diets in general, they are very healthy when done correctly, but in recovery I discourage people from dismissing foods or being vegetarian or vegan until recovered and able to eat all foods.

You can always go back to being vegetarian or vegan after making peace with food, but it is difficult to know if your food choices are for the right reasons until you have worked through your food issues.

Take this worksheet and come up with three meals per day for at least two different days based on things that you actually like and are willing to eat. They don't have to be things that you've eaten this week, but think about what's realistic and what actually interests you (you can rewrite meals as often as needed, as your food rules and portions loosen up). These meals can be things that you make at home, eat at a restaurant, or pick up at a cafeteria.

After coming up with meals, look at snacks. If you already have snacks you like, that's fine for now. Ideally, I would like you to work up to snacks that pair a carbohydrate with a protein or a fat, as those pairings are going to keep you full longer. I prefer that people are not having only a fruit or a vegetable as a snack, but rather pairing that with something else, like an apple with peanut butter. What other snack ideas can you come up with?

> ## Optimal macronutrient percentages as a percentage of overall (adequate) calorie intake
>
> Carbohydrates: about 45–65 percent
> Fats: about 20–35 percent
> Proteins: about 10–35 percent
>
> *Quick tip: Alcohol is the only other calorie-containing molecule, and the only one not required to live. If you drink, please drink responsibly and in moderation.

A word on diets and cleanses

Skip the diets, generic meal plans, and anything that encourages cutting out food groups. Our bodies are designed to eat a variety of foods, use nutrients, and do their own detoxification. You don't need to do a "detox" or "cleanse" EVER. You have a liver and kidneys that automatically do that for you. Pretty cool, right?

Dieting is the number one predictor of developing an eating disorder, especially among teens. There is also a number one way to prevent the development of an eating disorder—DON'T DIET. Healthy eating is actually pretty simple. Eat a variety of foods and let your body do the rest.

How much to eat

I'm going out on a limb here, but a question I get all the time is, "How much should I eat?" Unfortunately, there's not a simple answer. There are lots of different factors behind how much a person should eat. It varies depending on your activity level, body type, and can even depend on the day. So, I'm going to give you the basic requirements with the hope that you're going to work one-on-one with a registered dietitian to determine your unique needs.

Every mammal has what's called a resting metabolism. This is the number of calories we use daily just to keep our body alive and functioning. For example, if you were in a hospital bed in a coma, you would still require calories to keep your organs going. These include your heart, your lungs, your kidneys, your immune system, and your other organs, even if you're completely unaware of any of them. For most adults, the resting metabolic rate is around 1,200 to 1,500 Calories, with larger people needing a bit more. This is the absolute minimum that we need to be eating. Activity, brain function, healing, movement, and growth all require more calories on top of that. So, for most adults, we need a *minimum* of 1,500 Calories a day (sedentary), but most young adults need quite a bit more.

The diets I see in women's and fitness magazines are typically 1,500 to 1,600 Calories/day. This is definitely *not* enough for a teen or young adult (or most adults for that matter). At college age, a *minimum* of around 2,000 Calories is appropriate for (biological) females, and a *minimum* of about 2,400 Calories for (biological) males, and more if you are very active or have a faster metabolism. If you're growing, underweight, pregnant, very active or compete in sports, have a larger or taller body, you will need more. People who are recovering from major surgery or burn injuries require even more!

"Caloric Conundrum"

During the recovery from anorexia, it has been widely noted in studies that there is a period in refeeding where the metabolic needs are astronomical—as much as 4,000 to 8,000 Calories a day! This doesn't last forever, but it can be scary for people who have been eating so little for so long.

The term "caloric conundrum" was coined by Dr. Walter Kaye, who noted that at a certain point in restriction, it takes so little food to continue to lose weight but so much to gain even a few ounces.

With all that being said, I don't want this to turn into (or exacerbate) an obsession for you. So, **if you don't currently count calories, please don't start!** You don't need to. Our culture has become so obsessed with tracking numbers and data. Honestly, we don't need to do this except in very special cases.

Up until the 1990s, nutrition facts labels as we know them (with calories and numbers) were not mandatory and had only been recently introduced to the food industry. What did people do before? They didn't count! I think we can learn a lot from the history of how people ate. Meals were often eaten in community (with family or other groups) and were comprised of proteins, starches, and vegetables. Milk was served with most meals. While body image and weight loss resulted in other scary alternatives, calorie counting was not a part of it; food was just food.

Another way to create balanced meals

The USDA MyPlate was created to replace the confusing Food Pyramid and is an excellent example of what a balanced meal looks like (you can see it at choosemyplate.gov, or the more specific Harvard Healthy Eating Plate). The MyPlate model makes things a lot easier because there are no specific portion sizes. Still, it gives you a good visual representation of proportions, not portions, of food you should be eating at a given meal. Remember, not all meals need to look like this! We're not striving for perfection, but balance.

This model looks like having about three-quarters of our plate consist in carbohydrate-rich sources. Ideally, about half should come from produce, a quarter from grains or starch, and another quarter from sources of protein. Make sure to include a good source of calcium and some fat. If you're eating the majority of your meals this way, you're doing really well. If you pair this concept with the Rule of 3s plan, you know you're going to be hitting all of your bases and getting the nutrients you need.

Turning orange?

I'll never forget the first time I saw a client who pointed out that her palms and feet were looking darker than usual—and when I looked I saw they were actually turning orange! The cause is eating too many orange and yellow foods like carrots, sweet potatoes, and pumpkin.

Vitamin A (beta-carotene), which is responsible for yellow and orange coloring in foods, is a fat-soluble vitamin, meaning that it is stored in fat tissue in the body. It can build up in the body and turn you orange! This strange-looking phenomenon usually starts in and stays in the thicker areas of skin, like palms, knees, and bottoms of the feet, but can spread to all body tissue.

Luckily, this is relatively harmless and totally reversible by abstaining from these foods for a while, and then eating them in normal, instead of excessive, quantities.

Variety in the diet is key.

Eating zones

While you are learning your hunger and fullness cues, it can be helpful to have some structure to your day. Something my clients find useful is creating "eating zones," or chunks of time for a meal or snack. Between those zones are chunks of time during which you don't eat. Eating zones prevent grazing all day long and help you to notice hunger cues more easily.

For example: breakfast between 6 and 7AM, then nothing until snack time between 9 and 10AM, then a break until lunch between 12:30 to 1:30PM, etc. This should be based on your schedule and preferences. Eating zones give you quite a bit of flexibility, but you still need to eat in a way that ensures you're getting your needs met. These zones also free up brain space since you won't be obsessing over when you are going to eat next.

Strict eating zones should NOT be a lifelong thing, but this plan can help you develop the habit of spacing out food. It is especially useful for people who save all their eating until the end of the day, or those who graze all day long. As with all of the ideas in this book, please allow for flexibility. This can turn into a rigid, obsessive plan if not given space, and is definitely not for everyone.

Late-night eating

There is no magic cut-off time for eating. Your metabolism doesn't stop while you sleep. If you stay up late to do homework (or watch Netflix, no judgment), you might need a late-night snack to keep going.

To wrap up this section, we meet our nutrient and vitamin needs by choosing from a variety of macronutrients, colors, and types of foods. We also need to make sure that we eat foods we enjoy. Adding some structure to meal "planning" and timing can help you get back on track, but you need to remain flexible if you are using them.

Main takeaways:

- Foods are not good or bad. All foods fit in a healthy diet, and the less you avoid them, the less power they have over you. You have permission to eat what you like.
- Don't diet. Your body has natural hunger and fullness cues. Listen! These cues should bring your body to its natural "happy weight," which does not require work to maintain.
- Get proportions in order. We need all the macronutrients and need them in proportion with each other. Remember, carbs are the majority at roughly 45 to 65 percent of calories, proteins are 10 to 35 percent, and fats are 20 to 35 percent. You don't need to calculate this, it's just for reference.
- Space out your food over the course of the day rather than eating one or two meals.

Take action:

Download the meal planning worksheet.

Plan at least two days of different meals you could realistically try. Can you fill in all the categories?

Pick a new fruit or vegetable to try this week. What colors do you typically miss?

Are you eating enough based on the calorie minimums discussed in this chapter? How can you adjust?

If you struggle with spacing out your food, create "eating zones" that fit into your schedule.

Chapter 4

Rock Your Body (Image)

"Mother Teresa didn't walk around complaining about her thighs; she had shit to do."

—Sarah Silverman

Let's get real. Eating disorders are life-threatening illnesses, and we can help ourselves and others get better through our behaviors and words. We all need to do our part to stop the "fat talk." When we comment negatively about our own body, others hear it and start to question their own. What if we were actually nice to our bodies?

Diet culture is all around us, luring us in with claims of "losing 10 pounds in two weeks!" or "the superfood you are missing," or "hidden dangers in your fridge!"

Ugh. Fearmongering. The *Oxford English Dictionary* definition of fearmongering is: *"the action of deliberately arousing public fear or alarm about a particular issue."*

And boy, do marketing people know how to use this to their advantage! Unfortunately, this is used with food, supplements, diets, and programs ALL THE FREAKIN' TIME!

In general, if it sounds too good to be true, it probably is. A good rule I heard is if you are hearing about the magic pill/cure/food/diet that you have been missing on an afternoon talk show for the first time, it's not legit. We would have heard about it from reliable scientific sources first.

But I get it. I, too, have been drawn in by the siren song of a supplement or superfood that would "speed up metabolism" or other such claims, despite knowing better (that's embarrassing!). I am ashamed to say I have tried some of the so-called miracle supplements, like green coffee bean and garcinia cambogia. I remember wanting to lose a little more weight before my wedding (I look back at photos and I looked amazing without weight loss). The pills only lasted a week or so, as I felt like I had cotton stuck in my throat for hours after taking them. Needless to say, they didn't help me lose weight, just cash. I was lucky. Some of these diet pills can cause more serious problems than a light wallet. Some can be deadly!

When researching and selecting supplements, drugs, and other "natural cures," ask yourself:

- What is the purpose of the source (website, advertisement, article) you are getting the information from? Do they have a vested interest in selling or is it purely educational?
- Is your doctor/whoever getting kickback from the company to sell their product? What is their reason for recommending it? Practitioners, ethically, should not be direct sellers of supplements and medications. If they do sell them, they MUST allow you to purchase from anywhere you want, not just from them.
- Claims that are supported by scientific evidence are important! How big was the study(s)? Same demographic of people as yourself? Were the results actually significant? Was there a strong control or could the results be attributed to other lifestyle changes?
- "NSF," "USP," or "US Pharmacopeia" should be on the package of dietary supplements to indicate that standards of processing were followed for safety and that the product contains the ingredients it says it does. (Note: this does not necessarily mean that the dose or ingredients are safe to consume, effective, or necessary for humans at all.)
- "Natural" does not inherently equal "safe." Many toxic substances are "natural," like mercury and cocaine. We don't need to consume those! Many safe substances are man-made, like the life-saving medication Synthroid, used for thyroid disorders.

- Check the Office of Dietary Supplements for research-driven fact sheets about specific supplement substances (though it doesn't cover specific brand formulas, which, again, might not have what is listed). The website is: https://ods.od.nih.gov/.

Whether you choose to take supplements or not, do your research, be careful, and ask yourself if it is something you really need. Sometimes the answer will be yes (for deficiencies like calcium, vitamin D, or iron), and sometimes it will be a hell, no! (substances that may be harmful or unnecessary for humans like Coq10, saw palmetto, or Garcinia cambogia).

No weigh!

In all honesty, weight is not as important a health indicator as once thought. In fact, most health issues are independent of weight. Lifestyle plays a role, for sure, but not weight specifically. Research on health outcomes led to the awesome Health at Every Size® movement (HAES). HAES means that health is not measured by weight, and you (and your health professionals) can care for your body no matter what size body you have. We've seen blood sugars and cholesterol drop without weight loss, showing that weight loss is not the "cure-all" it was once thought to be. How we live has a much bigger impact on our health.

How much do you let the number on the scale dictate how your day is going to go? What if you let that go? If you're like me, the number was never "good enough." I never got off the scale feeling better about myself. When I stopped weighing myself, I was able to let the events of the day dictate my mood instead of a number that only reflected my gravitational pull to the earth. I threw out my scale and haven't seen my weight in over a year. And guess what? My clothes still fit! I didn't keep gaining weight (I know, mind blown!).

On that note, you have the right to not be weighed at the doctor's office, or to not see the number if you don't want to know. Tell the nurse before they make you hop on the scale. It can be useful for medical providers to monitor your weight if you are severely underweight, or for children still growing, but beyond that there is really no need. They can estimate for most medicinal needs.

Dangerous dieting

By now, it should be no surprise to you that I am not a fan of dieting. But why? So many people claim they work. Am I wrong? Let's look at what happens with a fad diet.

Why diets "work" (but not really)

There is a basic formula for any fad diet book you pull off the shelf:

1. Choose a "superfood"/ingredient/macronutrient to plug
2. Restrict other options (add a good dose of fear if you want to make it seem more exciting)
3. Get a celeb/influencer to endorse it

This same principle applies whether it is "low carb," "low fat," or no *X* foods. The magical weight loss formula doesn't have anything to do with the specific food or macronutrient. So why do they "work" in the short term?

The diet "works" by limiting favorite foods, which leads to decreased calories, resulting in short-term weight loss. This weight loss is caused by not having options of foods to eat, which gets boring and you end up eating less (the rest of the book reviews why this is not good in the long term). Or, the diet drastically limits carbohydrates (Keto, Atkins, Paleo, South Beach, etc.). Carbohydrate molecules attach to water molecules in our body, keeping us hydrated. When they are cut down, we experience a quick drop in water weight—the "lose six pounds in two days" scheme. It's NOT fat loss. The moment you eat carbs, you gain several pounds of water back, making you feel addicted to the diet. It's not healthy.

These diets inevitably backfire by:

1. Being so restrictive they cannot be maintained and the dieter "falls off the wagon" and feels shame (perhaps even binging on "forbidden foods").
2. Causing loss of water weight and muscle mass along with fat loss makes the body weaker, and not the lean and fit body composition the dieter was going for.
3. Jump-starting an eating disorder by creating distrust around bodily hunger cues.

Furthermore, weight cycling (when your weight goes up and down over and over, also called "yo-yo-dieting") is actually more harmful to our health than having always lived in a larger body. There are many factors to consider here, but the one you probably care about is that lowering calories for extended periods of time (from dieting or famine) causes our metabolism to lower forever! This means it will take fewer and fewer calories to maintain weight, let alone lose weight. This is actually a pretty cool adaptive response of our body. Our body wants to keep us alive! If it has to use fewer calories to do so, it will adapt. But for those working hard to diet and lose weight, it actually backfires. This is why people generally regain weight after a diet and find dieting harder and harder the more they do it.

Is recovery worth it? A thousand times, YES!!!

"Recovery can be a long, exhausting, infuriating, and devastating process—so you might be wondering why it's worth it. The answer is that living with an eating disorder is also long, exhausting, infuriating, and devastating. But unlike recovery, which is temporarily hard but incredibly rewarding, engaging with your eating disorder will hurt forever. No matter how much control you manage to exercise over your behaviors, it never gets better. I can guarantee that you won't actually be happy even if you reach your dream weight—how could you be, when you destroyed your health and used self-loathing as motivation in order to get there? To have an eating disorder is to stew in a pot of misery every day. You won't magically leap out of the misery pot and into the joy pot just because you stood on a square of plastic and electronics that handed you a different number in the morning.

When I was in my eating disorder, there were times when I was quite thin. Did I sometimes feel proud of my protruding clavicles? Sure. But I spent much more time feeling hungry, weak, shaky, headachy, sleep deprived, and irritable. All of the other things that I was passionate about fell by the wayside—I didn't have meaningful relationships or important goals beyond my eating disorder. I had to hide and lie and exercise until my joints screamed. I was a miserable shell of a person.

Today, I am at a healthy weight, and I can tell you with absolute certainty that what matters is not your body but the way you feel about it. When I was at this weight in my eating disorder, the hatred I felt for my body was indescribable. I thought nothing on earth could be more hideous than I was. I look exactly the same as I did back then, but now I am grateful for every part of my body, including the curve of my stomach after I eat, and the healthy layer of fat on my thighs. Nourishing my body with healthy (but not obsessive!) food and regular (but not obsessive!) exercise feels a thousand times better than the supposed satisfaction of a number on a scale. There are no downsides to recovery. None. Please join me on the other side and find the confidence and joy that await you here."

—Anonymous friend who has recovered from anorexia nervosa, binge-purge subtype

The "F-word"

Fat.

What a loaded word. With one utterance, it can bring someone's self-esteem crashing down. Let's unpack the meaning of the word "fat." The word "fat" in the context of degradation is referring to adipose tissue in the body. Adipose tissue is living body tissue. The fat cells have a nucleus and blood supply. They are metabolically active. While fat cells can get bigger than needed, they are essential to many bodily functions; but all you see is "fluff."

If we look further back in history to the ancient Greeks, the Renaissance period, and many other times in history, having curves, rolls, and some extra junk in the trunk was the height of beauty! The most famous artists of all time painted and sculpted the voluptuous figures that we still marvel at today. Over the course of history, what is in fashion in regard to body type changes every decade or so, filling in and out as the seasons change, like clothes in the stores. When voluptuous bodies were popular, those who were thin were put-down. In other cultures, even today, being slender is shameful, as it means you must be poor.

The truth is everyone has body fat. In fact, if we have none, we die. Fat is protective and cushions our organs and bones. It literally stores energy, but it is also responsible for much more. It is active in our nervous system as "insulation" for conductive neurons like electrical wire coverings. It is a major part of our endocrine system, responsible for storing and being part of the makeup of hormonal messengers, including leptin, which tells our brain to stop eating. It makes up a huge chunk of our brain matter. It regulates our temperature. Fat is essential.

By virtue of having fat, you have a functioning human body. It's normal. Hopefully, someday, "fat" will not be a put-down, but for now, know that those using it against you (or others) are really saying they are insecure about themselves and they know they can push your buttons with the "f-word." Don't let them get to you. You really are beautiful when YOU, and only you, are comfortable with your body.

Who are you without your label?

Do you define yourself by your eating or exercise habits? Are you labeled as the "health nut"? The "jock"? The "foodie"? The "thin one"? How much of your identity is wrapped up in your disorder?

Now, think of who you are without these labels. What else are you? What are your passions and strengths? Are you a painter? Good listener? Skilled musician? Reliable? If you are like a lot of my clients, this is an extremely difficult mental block. You've invested so much of yourself in your "health" (not-so-healthy health) labels, but know you are so much more than your disorder!

You are worthy of love and belonging, just as you are. Being thinner, faster, a better vegan, more *whatever* does not make you worthier.

Write a mantra in your journal and read it daily. Some ideas:

I am worthy just as I am.
I am lovable just as I am.
Different is beautiful.
My body does not define me.

Writing your why statement

One of the most powerful tools for motivation on the path to loving yourself is having a clearly defined "*why.*" This comes easier once you can identify who you are without your ED.

Why do you want to change? What does life look like without ED? What will you be able to do that you can't do while stuck in the abusive relationship with ED?

Write (or type) this out on nice paper. Carry it with you or post it where you will see it every day. This is easiest to write when you are feeling motivated and strong, and most necessary to read when you are feeling weak and powerless. You have the ability to change your life. You can make big changes or small changes. Every choice can move you forward or leave you in your current situation. What choice do you want to make today?

What have some of my other clients written as their "why" statements?

Maddie's "why"

"I want to recover because I want to spend more time appreciating and enjoying my food rather than weighing and measuring it with obsessive precision.

I want to recover because I want to melt into the warmth of my lover's embrace instead of resisting it with numb indifference.

I want to recover because I want the energy to be emphatically expressive like the proud Italian I am.

I want to recover because I want to take delight in the wet kisses of an enthusiastic dog.

I want to recover because I want to belly laugh until I can't breathe and sob until I have no tears left.

I want to recover because I want to sing at the top of my lungs to my favorite songs and succumb to the masterful flow of beautiful music.

I want to recover because I want to receive a hand-prepared, traditional meal from a foreign host, and think only of the generosity bestowed instead of worrying over calories and ingredients.

I want to recover because I want the vitality to carry me through long flights, jet lag, and days filled with sightseeing on foot.

I want to recover because I want the strength to scale mountains and help a neighbor move in their furniture, and tussle on the floor with a pet.

I want to recover because I want the clarity of mind to focus on the words of a loved one, to really listen and hear and remember.

I want to recover because I want to help other people like me, who have suffered as I have, and I want to show them what is possible.

I have a thousand reasons why, but above all else I want to recover because I want to live."

(Used with permission.)

"I want to follow my meal plan right now because this is going to help me get to the things I cannot imagine life without [that won't be possible with ED in the way]."

—Anonymous client

Some other reasons my clients have given:

- Be in a healthy relationship with someone else
- Have a social life
- Be able to travel
- Be confident
- Be able to exercise and be active
- To think clearly and have better memory
- Feel my emotions/feelings
- Write a book on my experiences
- Help other people
- Have a career

What is your why?

"If you have a big enough WHY, you will figure out the how."
—*Tony Robbins*

> ### What I learned from drag queens
>
> My good friend, who stage manages the local drag shows, gave me a fantastic opportunity to help out with drag events and have a blast hanging out with the queens in the dressing room. And can they teach us all a thing or two about body acceptance!
>
> For those who don't know, a drag queen is someone (most often a man, but can be any gender) who dresses up in women's clothes (usually gowns and over-the-top makeup, complete with huge false eyelashes—but drag "kings" are also a thing), typically for purposes of entertainment (e.g. drag show).
>
> As I watched these queens get ready, I noticed several things that I think we can take away from the experience:
>
> 1. Curves. Many of the queens actually add padding to accentuate curves. They add hips and breast, and it is not in jest. They genuinely think this is beautiful. How many of us have tried to hide our feminine form? To starve or run off the curves? The queens would be appalled. Takeaway: rock the curves you were given.
>
> 2. They take up space. Even when getting ready, the world is their stage. The tables, floor, and every surface is "theirs"— they don't try to contain their fabulousness. It almost seems a point of pride to have more space and to drive out another queen (though the locals here tend to get along well and help each other out). Takeaway: it is okay to take up space!

3. They are unapologetic in how they present. Queens don't shuffle along with heads hung low trying to disappear, they f-ing shine! A queen sashays in her stilettos, head up, shoulders back, checking that her lipstick is on point. She does not apologize for being there, being the center of attention, or walking in front of you. Takeaway: Hold your head up proudly, walk confidently, and as Coco Chanel said, "If you are sad, add more lipstick and attack!"

Main takeaways:

- Watch out for quacks and unnecessary health products. Do your research before trying supplements or other products/plans!
- You are worthy. Right here. Right now.
- Losing weight will not make you happier/make people like you.
- Fat is an essential part of our body's function.
- It's okay to take up space.

Take action (grab your journal):

Write your "why" statement for recovery. What does future you get to do that is not possible if you stay in your disorder? Who are you without ED?

Write out a recovery mantra. For example: "I am worthy right now, and I have permission to eat."

Think of one way you can live a little more like a drag queen (and I am not saying you need to load on the makeup if that is not you!). How can you stand confidently in a room? What will it take to look up instead of at your feet? What clothes make you feel fabulous in your current body? Wear them!

Watch Amy Cuddy's TED Talk on gaining confidence with power poses:

https://www.ted.com/talks/amy_cuddy_your_body_language_shapes_who_you_are?utm_campaign=tedspread&utm_medium=referral&utm_source=tedcomshare

Get rid of your home scale and work/school scales if possible. If you can, smash them. It is a very cathartic way to symbolize your newfound freedom.

Chapter 5

How To Actually Stop Behaviors

"There is a difference between interest and commitment. When you are interested in something you do it only when it is convenient. When you are committed to something, you accept no excuses; only results."

—Kenneth Blanchard

This chapter is designed to give you more actionable ideas for working on your specific behaviors. Feel free to skip the sections that don't apply to you or read it all and help a friend. They all take work and commitment, but if you stick it out, you will develop the tools you need to change your relationship with food.

Meeting a craving

Have you ever done this?

A warm pan of brownies is cooling. They look amazing. Fudgy and fresh. I could have a small one. No. I'm going to "be good," I'll have some carrots instead. Damn, the brownies still sound so good. Okay, it's dinner time, I'll eat a balanced dinner. Still want the brownie. I'll have an apple instead. That is still not satisfying the desire for the brownie. It's now late and I've been battling this craving all day. I eat half of the pan of brownies. I feel sick, and worse, ashamed. I should have been stronger than the siren call of the brownies.

This used to be a frequent occurrence for me until I learned how to just eat the brownie when I first wanted it. I learned that if I ate a food I craved when I first craved it, this pattern stopped completely. I've explained this thought pattern to many clients who all nod, wide-eyed at me. *Yes, yes, this happens All. The. Time.* When they try eating the craved food up-front, they are amazed by their ability to eat a reasonable portion and leave the rest.

Eating this way is eating intuitively. Intuitive eating means listening to, and trusting, your body. It's not just about hunger and fullness (though that is definitely part of it), it's also about listening to what your body wants and needs. A lot of people are afraid if they eat whatever they are craving, they will just eat "junk" food, but our body doesn't want that all the time. If we truly listen, our body will also crave vegetables and other types of foods.

After years of mistrust, it can be a lot to trust your body. But I promise, not only is it so worth it, it actually makes life so much easier! I no longer worry how many calories I am eating, or if I am eating "healthy" enough. I trust that my body will balance it out for me. Health is an ongoing process. Our body doesn't reset every night at midnight. One "bad" day or meal is not a deal breaker. Strive for balance over the week, rather than having "perfect" days.

Quick tip: If you struggle with "safe" versus "unsafe" foods (maybe you call them something else like "good" versus "bad" foods) that you are trying to reincorporate into your diet, save the "safe" foods for the end of the meal so you get the others in.

One way to stop binge eating

I was an extremely lucky kid. An only child, I was respected by my parents. An example that comes to mind was when one of us had a "special" food that we loved, we could tell the others (or put a note on it) that it was ours, and the other two wouldn't touch it. For example, my Halloween candy would go into a Tupperware with my name on it, and they wouldn't touch it unless I offered it. This candy could last nine months (!) or more because there was no urgency to eat it.

Moving on to college, I never really shared food with roommates. We bought our own stuff, and unless we had a huge surplus that we decided to share, we just stayed in our respective lanes. So it was quite the wake-up call when I got married and all of a sudden I was sharing food with my husband. This may have been the most difficult part of living with another person.

One distinct memory I have from my first year of marriage was buying a pumpkin pie. I had a slice and covered the rest up for later. About two days later, I decided I wanted another slice and lifted the lid to find that the whole pie was nearly gone (to clarify, my husband is not a binge eater, just a hungry man without body image issues)! I frantically ate the remainder of the pie, worried that if I didn't I wouldn't get any more. Eventually, I bought another pie and in anticipation that it might happen again, I ate more than I was hungry for. Between the two of us, we finished that large Costco pie in about two days. The pattern repeated with lots of foods in the house for over a year. I was miserable. I gained about 20 pounds that year, was anxious, and seriously rethinking my living arrangement.

At some point, I realized there will always be more food. You can buy more, make more, ask your aunt for the recipe, find a new food you love. You don't have to eat it all this second. When I really wanted something, I went and got more. If it was all gone in the morning and I didn't get as much as I wanted, I bought or made more. By simply having the food around, I reduced the urgency of eating it and was able to decide if I really wanted it or how much I wanted. It was so freeing.

Why you binge

There are three main reasons binge eating develops.

1. **Deprivation-driven overeating:** dieting or saying you "can't have x food" = obsessed with eating what is "scarce" = overeating when you get the chance.
2. **Self-medicating:** happens when you feel numb or comforted from eating too much; it can lead to self-loathing (shame).
3. **Habitual overeating:** Neglecting body signals of hunger/fullness over time leads to developing a habit of eating the way you trained yourself to eat. This can come from family eating patterns, environment (e.g. free food at work), or other sources.

How to apply this to yourself:

If you struggle with binging, I've got a tried-and-true tactic for neutralizing binge trigger foods: You're going to eat a trigger food on a regular basis.

Take a moment and let that sink in. Don't get too anxious, we're going to do it in a way that will make the food lose power over you, for good.

Scarcity and deprivation create a sense of urgency (think of marketing tactics like "only two left in stock!"). So, when we have access to something that we have deprived ourselves of enjoying, it is human nature to overeat it. Before you try this method, you

MUST commit to following through. I have seen this work well for a lot of people when they commit. However, if you get scared and give up, you can end up with a worsened relationship with food. Proceed at your own risk.

Note: Binge cessation is usually not a "cold turkey" stop. Normally, it becomes less and less frequent with time. Don't beat yourself up if you have a lapse. Every day you don't binge or do another ED behavior is a win!

The plan: Pick one binge-trigger food that you love, but don't normally allow yourself. Buy (or make) a "family-size" amount (large bag, many servings). Pick only one food and be very specific about flavor, brand, etc.

Allow yourself to eat this food as fast as it naturally happens. Don't force-feed, but don't restrict either. The first day or few days, most people will binge on it. As scary as it is, allow this to happen if it naturally does. As soon as you run out or run low on the food, go buy more of the exact same food (same flavor, brand, etc.). This is important. Continue the process of eating. The goal here is to make this food less scarce, less urgent. When we stop depriving ourselves of something, we actually have *more* control. When you can keep the food in the house for several days and you don't feel compelled to binge on it, you have completed the exercise. This has taken my clients, on average, two to four weeks. Once you have completed this with one specific food, choose another food and repeat as needed. This should go much faster. Most people only need to do this with one or two foods to get to the point of decreased urgency with all food.

Emotional overeating

For many, binging or overeating is emotionally numbing or self-soothing. If this is what you struggle with, I have a different approach. Are you finding that you turn to food when you are very stressed or emotional as a way to numb whatever is going on in your life? I'm sorry to tell you, but food is not going to fix the situation. When you are numbing out, you are not changing your situation.

Ultimately, you need to take action that will create peace around the situation. This might mean having a difficult conversation to resolve an issue; or it may be a more drastic life change like quitting a job, getting out of a relationship, finding a new friend group, or moving. If that is not immediately possible (logistically, mentally, or safely), look for healthier coping mechanisms. I cover a few in chapter 7.

What is the hardest thing about recovery?

"Having to actively choose to override your hardwired brain chemistry and negative habits. You have to deliberately decide to go against what you believed to be normal and trust that you can have freedom and a better life."

—Recently recovered young woman

Regardless of why you overeat or binge eat, the best way to prevent future binges is to stay on a normal eating schedule. If you binge, **make sure to eat your next scheduled meal or snack.** Remember the binge-restrict cycle from chapter 1? Being hungry is a self-fulfilling binge prophecy.

Purging

Self-induced vomiting is a strange behavior. People who don't do it will never understand why you would voluntarily throw up. It feels icky!

But if you do it, there is a reason. It feels momentarily calming and gives you a sense of control. There is literally a physiologically calming chemical rush when vomiting (whether from the flu, food poisoning, or eating disorder), but it is short lived. In the ED, there is also the mental rush that you "got rid of" what you ate. It feels "clean."

Sorry to tell ya, but it actually doesn't get rid of the majority of your food. Some common myths with purging:

Myth: It gets rid of most of your calories.

Reality: Nope! Evidence by Dr. Walter Kaye has shown that the majority of calories are retained once they hit the stomach. In binge to purge, at least 1,200 Calories are retained! Our body is very efficient at grabbing nutrients, especially if we don't eat enough on a regular basis.

Myth: You see your food come up in the reverse order it went down.

Reality: Nope! A lot of people use "marker" foods, brightly colored foods like beets or salad, to try to show when they have gotten everything up. Well, it doesn't work that way. Food gets all mixed up as soon as it goes in, so colors are not going to tell you how much is left in your stomach.

Myth: You should brush your teeth after purging.

Reality: Please don't! Brushing immediately after vomiting (even when you have the flu) is a bad idea, as you are actually rubbing the stomach acids into your teeth and further damaging the enamel. Instead of brushing, wait at least an hour, swish and spit with water, and if you can, add a pinch of baking soda (not baking powder, which has acid in it) to the mouthful of water. The higher pH of the baking soda helps to neutralize the low pH of stomach acid.

Vomiting can cause big problems, including systemic infection! Mallory-Weiss tears are open wounds in the lining of the esophagus, which will show up as pain when vomiting or acid reflux occurs. You will likely see red blood in your vomit. If you see blood, go to urgent care! Since this is an open wound, you can get infected just as if you had a cut on the outside of your body. With food and acid flowing over the tears, you can get bacteria into your bloodstream, which can cause major problems like sepsis (full body infection that is hard to treat). Additionally, if you take medications, vomiting within two to three hours of taking them can prevent absorption, rendering them mostly useless.

Steps to help you stop self-induced vomiting:

Delay, Delay, Delay! If you can put off a purge for a while, you are less likely to go through with it. Start with 10 or 15 minutes and work up to eventually not needing to purge at all. Purging is a coping behavior, and if you can delay it by doing something distracting and nonharmful, you can train yourself to not need it. Go for a walk, talk to a friend, and stay out of the bathroom after eating. See chapter 7 for more examples.

It can also be very helpful to track when you are binging and purging. You can mark this on your food and feelings journal (chapter 2) with a "B" or "P" to keep it simple. Look back at what situations lead to purges. Is it related to certain situations (when no one is home or after eating out) or emotional triggers? By noting your triggers, you can focus on delaying or other strategies, such as staying out of the bathroom for an hour after eating.

If you use any "tools" to help you vomit (e.g. toothbrush, swallowing something), stay away from them (and the bathroom) after eating or when you feel triggered. Better still, get rid of them altogether (keep the toothbrush but pay attention to use).

When you do vomit, swallow it back. Instead of letting the vomit out of your mouth, keep it in and swallow. Disgusting, I know, but this is pretty effective at breaking the habit.

Chewing and spitting

This is a behavior that can almost be completely resolved by looking at why you are using the behavior. Most people who chew and spit (CHSP) primarily restrict intake and tend to CHSP when feeling out of control (70 percent based on a 2015 study). CHSP does not do much in terms of weight loss, and instead creates a worse relationship with food and undermines your ability to trust yourself. What's more, it often leads to cavities and other dental problems as a result of the extended amount of time that your teeth are coated in food.

Mindful eating (covered later in this chapter) is a big help in reducing CHSP. Know that CHSP is a form of restricting, binging, and purging all in one! Try to abstain from buying large packages of foods that you CHSP. Instead, focus on eating small portions of "scary" foods, slowly building up to more. You will find that nothing bad happens when you actually eat the food, and it is a lot more satisfying (and less urgent) to eat knowing you don't have to spit it out.

How to stop using laxatives, diuretics, and diet pills

Laxatives are dangerous for your body, just like vomiting. They throw off electrolytes, dehydrate you, and can cause serious long-term G.I. issues from using them to poop. It is easier on your body to cut back laxatives over time rather than stop cold turkey; unless you are taking a low dose (one to two per day), in which case you can go ahead and stop cold turkey. If you are taking higher doses, cut back by half the amount every few days. Doing this helps with lessening constipation (which is normal to experience for a while) during the weaning-off period. It can also help to focus on slowly increasing fibrous foods and water in your diet.

Diuretics really only make you dehydrated. Any "weight loss" is strictly water weight (and electrolytes), not calories, and is quickly regained. Overuse of diuretics can screw up your body's natural fluid-balance mechanisms. A pint of water is equal to a pound. So, every pound you "lose" is really just two cups of water and hurtful to your body. You can stop taking diuretics and diet pills cold turkey. It may take a few days or weeks for your body to regulate after using diuretics for a long time. It is recommended that you see a medical professional when using diuretics, as long-term use (or for certain individuals in general) can cause kidney damage.

Most "diet pills," drugs, or supplements are either designed to speed up your metabolism with amphetamine ("speed") or similar drugs, to decrease natural appetite, or to drop water weight as with diuretics. Most diet drugs have been banned in many countries, which should tell us something. If they are "dietary supplements," they lack federal regulation that medications have and are not required to go through safety testing to be on the market. Others are off-label medications, which should only be used for their prescribed purpose (e.g. Adderall for ADHD) and not for weight loss. Just say no to diet pills.

With laxatives, diuretics, or diet pills, you may notice what appears to be "rebound weight gain," or feelings of "puffiness." Rest assured that it's just fluid (edema) between your cells that should go away on its own over a few weeks. If it is still not better in three weeks or so, go to your medical provider and tell them what is happening. Once you have stopped laxatives, diuretics, or diet pills, get rid of the rest! Take them to the garbage, drop them off at medicine disposal sites (at most pharmacies and some school health centers), or give them to someone else to get rid of for you. Just let that sh*t go.

Quick tip: If you feel full easily, save liquids until after you finish a meal (and try not to drink much 30 minutes before a meal to save room for the food).

Stop counting calories! Yes, it can be done[3]

If you are in the living hell of having the calorie counter constantly ticking in your head, then read on. This is one of the hardest things to break because even if you stop writing down or tracking in an app, your brain will continue to tally up food. Ugh!

I have a method that I successfully used for myself and many of my clients to stop counting. It is frustrating, but it works. The concept is simple: eat foods you can't accurately count. This means eating foods that are not individually packaged or easy to parse out into serving sizes. For instance, a turkey sandwich is easy to count because you can see (and measure) all the components. A casserole like lasagna would be hard to count; how much cheese, sauce, and noodle are you actually getting? It helps to have other people cook for you or to eat at restaurants (without calorie listings).

I told you it would be frustrating. You will probably get mad, cry, and want to go back to eating things that are easy to count or that you already know. Don't. Even if you start with one meal per day that you can't count, it is a good start. That's because it prevents you from having an accurate daily total. And if it's not accurate, what's the point? Keep this up, and eventually you will stop counting most foods because it ends up not being worth it. Then you are free!

---

3 You don't have to do this if you know you will not eat enough without counting. Work up to it once you can effectively take in enough calories. The end goal is to not have to count, but eating enough takes top priority.

★ Mindful eating exercise

Rooted in Buddhist Zen practices, mindfulness and mindful eating are getting a modern moment as we focus on trusting our internal feedback. This involves the use of all our senses: touch, taste, smell, sound, and sight. Whatever your food relationship, you can benefit from mindfulness practice. It can help you to appreciate your food on a much deeper level.

I've created a guided mindful eating exercise for you. You can read it below or listen to the audio version I have recorded for you at https://learn-with-libby.teachable.com/p/permission-to-eat. This is meant to be done slowly and deliberately. Do this exercise when you have at least 10 minutes and set the mood with quiet or soothing meditation music.

You are going to need a small snack. Typically, this experience is done with something like a raisin, a nut, or a small piece of chocolate, but you can use any food you have available.

Now that you have your food, we're going to have an experience with it. So, please don't eat it yet. We'll get to that point. Sit comfortably and let's begin. (This is where you can begin the mindful eating meditation recording if you are listening.)

First, I want you to hold the food in your hand and look at it. What are you seeing? Is it smooth? What color is it? Are there ridges? What colors do you see throughout the food? What else do you notice?

Just take a moment and look at all the different facets it encompasses. What does it feel like to hold in your hand? Is it sticky? Is it smooth and silky? Is it rough or grainy? Is it sharp? Recognize all the different textures in your food.

Now, I want you to take a big inhale and smell the food. What scents are you noticing? Is it fruity? Does it smell salty? Does it bring up memories for you? Maybe it was a positive childhood snack that you had.

Next, close your eyes. Take a big sniff again. Did it change? Are you more in tune with it? When we close off one sense, others are heightened.

Think about where this food came from. Did it grow from the ground? Did someone make it? What went into that process? Take a moment and just appreciate where it came from.

Now, without chewing, I want you to put it in your mouth. Don't eat it yet. Just set it on your tongue. What do you feel with your tongue? Is it sweet, bitter, salty, umami?

Now, I want you to chew it, just don't swallow it yet. What changed as you chew it? Are new flavors popping up? Does the texture change as you chew? Is it silky? Is it rough? Dry or juicy? What does it feel like in your mouth?

Finally, I want you to swallow it when you're done chewing. What flavors remain in your mouth? What lingers? Is it different?

I hope you'll try this exercise with a few different foods to see all the different textures, flavors, and other qualities you notice. This is something that we can apply to any meal or snack that we eat, though I don't expect you to have the time to do it every time you eat.

When you eat your regular meals and snacks, take time to really think about the flavors, textures, and smells that you're experiencing. Where did the food come from? Was it lovingly prepared? How did it grow? The more we appreciate our food, the better the relationship we can have with our food. Please take the time to do this exercise as many times as you need, and whenever you need a refresher.

Celebrating the small wins (something for everyone)

Celebrating accomplishments, however small, is an important skill in recovery and in life. This is not something I really understood as a perfectionist, that is until recently.

Throughout my life, I have been a goal-setter and achiever. Each December, for as long as I can remember, I would write out my big goals for the next year on a pretty piece of paper and post it in my room, so I'd see it every day. I have always achieved at least 80 percent of these goals by each year's end. I hadn't really thought about how I achieved these goals. I just knew they were important and took steps to make them happen. Still, throughout the year I struggled along, beating myself up for taking so long to reach the biggest of the goals. It is not often a linear path to achieving goals, as I'm sure you know. Whether it is recovering from an eating disorder, meeting an income goal, or being able to execute a dance move, goals take work.

In college, I stumbled into minoring in leadership. One of the classes we were required to take spent a lot of time celebrating accomplishments as they happened—not just year-end, big project goals, but little things. It was a form of team leadership, but we also had to apply it personally. This was really hard for me to wrap my head around at 20 years old. It is easy to celebrate a major win. 100 days binge-purge free. Graduating. Getting the lead in a play. These are major accomplishments. But when we are stuck in the minutiae of daily life, it is even more important to celebrate the small accomplishments. One day behavior free. Finished writing a paper. Made it through a family meal without crying. A week without suicidal thoughts. Able to go to a grocery store and actually purchase food in a reasonable amount of time.

These little wins are progress! Essential progress towards your larger goal. The importance of these wins is clear to me whenever I counsel my clients through recovery. I feel so privileged to see the big picture of their growth over the weeks and months while they are in the struggle of the day-to-day.

Recently, I was in a session with a client who was really struggling to see the "light at the end of the tunnel." She felt like she had been stuck in the eating disorder for so long. My heart hurt for her. She couldn't see the amazing work she had been doing over the past year we had been together. By taking a bird's-eye view of her progress, she was able to see that not only was she no longer suicidal (a huge improvement in itself!), she had been able to eat a much larger variety of foods (even though there are still some fear foods), her blood work had improved, and she was more social and had friends. A year before that would have terrified her.

She is not yet fully recovered. But no one can say that is not amazing progress!

I now ask many of my clients to keep an accomplishment log from week-to-week. It can be the smallest things like eating a certain food, or bigger things like going to a social event that felt scary. They don't have to show me, or anyone else, their log if they don't want to do so. The more we can own our accomplishments the more trust we have in ourselves to keep going, keep accomplishing, and build the skills we need to reach bigger goals. Success begets success.

Main takeaways:

- Action steps to help you stop calorie counting, overeating, or purging.
- Stay present with the practice of eating mindfully.
- Make sure to celebrate progress, no matter how small.

Take action (grab your journal):

Use the tips in the relevant sections of this chapter for what you need. Once you try something, journal about it. What feelings came up?

Try the mindful eating exercise.

Start writing down your successes each day or week. It may feel stupid at the time, but when you look back months or years from now, you will see how far you have come and feel more capable of making changes in the future.

Re-read your "why" statement.

Chapter 6

Wise Exercise

"You only have one body and despite how well you live your life, it may never change. Can you afford to hate yourself for the rest of your life?"

—Linda Bacon, *Health at Every Size*

Food issues don't occur in isolation. Often, exercise becomes a factor in trying to create control or regulate emotions. For many people, this looks like exercising too much or doing more than their weakened heart muscles can handle. For others, it is an avoidance of the gym or movement because of depression or a fear of being seen. It may be making sure to hit a certain time or calorie count on the machine (this can be eating disorder or OCD-related) or the rest of their day is ruined.

This doesn't have to be you.

I get it, we all want to look good and feel sexy and confident. I know I do, but there has to be a balance. We cannot push our "earth suits" to the point of damaging our body or soul.

Have you ever said no to really fun plans because you "had to" work out? When exercise becomes inflexible (I'm not talking about team practices for sports), you can be sure there is something deeper going on. One study from 2008 concluded that up to 42 percent of Parisian gym-goers had "a destructive relationship with exercise." Can you imagine how much worse that is today, over 10 years later, with all the fitness trends, and in America (versus France) where fitness and gym memberships are more mainstream? Yikes!

Fitspo & filters

Excessive exercise is a common form of compensation (a.k.a. purging) for eating among people with EDs. In fact, between 40 and 80 percent of people with anorexia nervosa excessively exercise as a means to avoid weight gain. This number may be even higher among those with bulimia nervosa!

This is not helped by trendy "fitspo" ("fitness-inspiration") posts that are rampant on the internet. It's not only not enough to be thin now, but you must also be insanely fit and muscular. This is often under the guise of "health," "wellness," and "getting strong," but it's really diet culture telling you your body is not good enough.

Along with fitness quotes about "no excuses," there is the rise in photography technology. We aren't limited to rudimentary Photoshop for professionals anymore. Now, there is advanced Photoshop for everyone, as well as Instagram filters and retouching apps. Whether altered or not, people tend to post the "highlight reel" of their lives online. Heck, even I do that (though I don't retouch my photos). Gone are the days of waiting until film was developed to toss out "bad" photos. We can take hundreds on a digital camera or smartphone to get one perfect photo that will still get retouched.

What can you do? If you are unable or unwilling to delete social media in general, at very least do yourself a favor and unfriend and unfollow any page that makes you feel bad about yourself. Life is too short to have a barrage of photos that make you hate yourself every time you open your phone. Follow accounts that make you smile. Friends that are posting real life, not just the retouched stuff. Photos of your hobbies or cute animals. There's something on the internet for everyone.

A primer on nutrition for fitness

Remember the ranges of macronutrients we talked about in chapter 2? These are ranges for a reason, and where you need to be depends on several factors including the types of activities you engage in. An endurance athlete will need more carbohydrates and less fat and protein than a weightlifter, who will need more protein and less carbohydrates (individual needs vary, and ideally are assessed by a RD). These do not (and should not) be taken to extremes. No matter your main type of activity, your body needs all three macronutrients within standard ranges, and a good variety of food to get all the micronutrients.

Your base calorie needs also increase as your activity level increases. Not only are you using more energy to move more, but as you gain more muscle you use more energy at rest! Muscle is more metabolically active (all day long) than adipose tissue, so as you get stronger, you also need to eat more. Something that many diet programs fail to mention is that when we lose weight we do not exclusively lose fat. Muscle is also lost, which accounts for a drop in metabolism.

Get moving

If you are not currently an active person, with some exceptions (like medically fragile low weight), movement is a good thing to do on a daily basis. It doesn't have to be long and hard. Let me share some of the things I learned during the eight years I was a personal trainer.

There are three necessary categories of movement: cardiovascular (aerobic and anaerobic), strength, and flexibility. This may be a review, but cardiovascular exercise primarily acts on the cardiorespiratory system (heart and lungs). Aerobic exercise literally means "with oxygen" and occurs during lower-intensity movement (walking, jogging, dance, paddle-boarding) and can be sustained for longer periods of time because our body can keep up with the need for oxygen in the cells. Anaerobic exercise "without oxygen" is done in short bursts of power movement (sprint, power lift, jump) and is not able to be sustained for long periods because the demand for oxygen cannot be met. Both are good for our heart and body (assuming you are healthy enough to do so).

Strength refers to any movement of the body or objects that uses skeletal muscles. Traditionally, people think of weightlifting, but strength training can be more functional with body resistance (think pushups, squats, planks) or daily tasks (pushing a cart, carrying groceries). For best results, give muscles a day off between strength activities to allow for tissue repair, which helps you gain muscle mass and avoid injury.

Flexibility is the unsung hero of fitness. Flexibility and balance are what will take you further in your sport and life. When we stretch, we are allowing the muscles to be more limber, thus reducing the risk of injury and making movement easier. Balance and flexibility are reasons that many elderly people fall and break bones. If you practice both on a regular basis, you are going to have much better quality of life as you age.

ED exercise complications

There are some particularly scary complications of excessive exercise (with or without an eating disorder). The main ones that concern me are: sudden cardiac death (more on this in chapter 9), amenorrhea, relative energy deficiency in sport, and bone fractures or breaks.

Sudden cardiac death

Anorexia nervosa has the highest death rate of any psychiatric illness and primarily from sudden cardiac death, which means your heart stops working. This is because there are not enough calories, either because you are not eating enough in general, or not eating enough for your activity level (even if you eat "normally"). Over time, organs, including the heart, lose function and energy supply. Malnourishment can be a ticking time bomb for the heart to stop completely. Don't be a statistic.

The first sign that the heart is suffering is a slowing down of your resting heart rate. Normal, healthy resting heart rate is 60 to 99 beats per minute (on the lower end for athletes). Once you are getting below about 45 bpm, please, please go to your physician and tell them what is going on. You may be thinking, "I'm an athlete, that's why my heart rate is low," but this can be a false sense of security if you are not fueling properly. Don't let pride or naiveté take you to the point of serious problems.

Female Athlete Triad/Relative Energy Deficiency in Sport (RED-S)

Well, despite the name having "female" in it, this diagnosis can affect all genders, hence the newer name "Relative Energy Deficiency in Sport." Thankfully, I have never heard anyone use the acronym for the triad because that would be unfortunate—F. A. T. (yikes!)

The "triad" is comprised of three traits someone with a uterus must have to be diagnosed. These are:

1. Amenorrhea—the absence of a menstrual period (obviously not a requirement for cis-males).
2. Not eating enough to meet energy needs (with or without body image concerns).
3. Decreased bone mineral density—the bones become more porous and likely to break when hormones and nutrition are off.

This issue primarily occurs with athletes (hence the name) in sports that value a lean physique such as running, ballet, and gymnastics. Although body dissatisfaction is not a requirement (this problem can come from a lack of nutrition education or access to food), the triad often occurs in tandem with an eating disorder. Research in 2012 found that 16 to 47 percent of elite female athletes had diagnosable eating disorders! That is higher than the national average for college-age females at 10 to 13 percent.

Treatment for RED-S is primarily about increasing energy availability by eating more calories (notice a trend in treatments?) and ensuring there is enough vitamin D, calcium, and other trace minerals to promote optimal bone density. A consistent return of menstrual periods often indicates improvement. Although many people with a uterus use birth control for this purpose, if the body is not doing this on its own, using hormonal contraceptives often creates a fake period and may mask issues like bone loss and malnutrition. Therefore, using hormones to induce a period is not recommended. Birth control should absolutely be used if needed for birth control—you can still get pregnant even if you are not menstruating—but it can cause a "false period" that does not mean you are healthy.

Why does it matter if you get a period at all? It's so nice to not worry about bleeding, amiright? Well, when your body does not create a menstrual cycle naturally, the lack of estrogen slowly makes bones less dense and more susceptible to breaks, fractures, and long-term osteoporosis and osteopenia. Long-term birth control like IUDs (intrauterine devices) don't appear to have any negative effects. Bone density scans have shown young people with the bone density of 80-year-olds! Lack of hormones can also cause growth to stop, resulting in adults who have the bone strength and stature of a child! Once you lose bone density, you can't get it back after your mid to late 20s, when new bone growth slows. After that, you are just working to maintain it. The gold standard for checking bone density is a DEXA/DXA (dual-energy X-ray absorptiometry) scan. Dr. Jennifer Gaudiani (the Gaudiani Clinic) has great information about it in her book *Sick Enough*.

Missing period? It's not a simple issue

"There is a natural ebb and flow in nature. In me, it is made of emotions and moons, of blood and tides.

When I first got my period at 11 years old, my mom baked me a red velvet cake. I was told it was a celebration, a welcoming to the sisterhood. The sisterhood is powerful. She helped me embrace my womanhood and told me to never be embarrassed of my period. She told me that every cramp, every cry, every moment of my cycle is felt by other women, and that this is the bond that connects us so tightly.

I watch the moon rise more often than the sunset, I see the waters breathe into the horizon.

When I first skipped my period at 19 years old, my mom wasn't too worried. This wasn't too out of the ordinary. I had just moved back home from college and imagined stress caused a skip. Then I missed another month, then another. Before I had even thought about it, six months passed without

---

an ounce of blood. I was worried, as were the women close to me, so I went to a doctor. The doctor assured me it was probably just a matter of stress from moving home. She dismissed my loss of periods to focus on a fracture in my foot from increased running.

I looked out into the strangely calm seascape. No waves crashed upon the shore.

I moved back to college. Another three months passed without my cycle before I saw another doctor. She recognized my lack of period that also came with an increase in exercise and weight loss. She tested my thyroids, hormones, and blood cell counts. All came back normal. That's when I was first diagnosed with an eating disorder.

Thunder rolls in the distance, water spouts sprout from the dark depths of the water, but the ocean is still and warm.

As it was explained to me, I wasn't eating enough and I was working out too much. My body couldn't support another life because it was struggling to support mine. My ovulation ceased. As time went on without my having a period, I felt an inner distance growing between myself and the women around me.

The tide continues to crawl away from me, the once wet sand has become arid and dry.

Many women loathe their periods. It's expensive, a hassle, uncomfortable. However, when you don't get periods, it feels the same—uncomfortable. I could always rely on my period before, something that happened monthly as a reminder that I was in good health, that my body was powerful enough to make another body. I don't like being told that I can't do something. I don't like feeling like I am not able, not powerful, not a part of the sisterhood.

My eyes dart for the moon in the sky, but it is covered by the blackness of the sky.

I still don't get my period. I have been recovered and weight stable for years and my period still hasn't returned. Some doctors say it is still from overexertion or stress, and not to worry about it. I have had to teach myself the core of sisterhood is not just biological—it is emotional. Without that physical reminder, I have to remind myself that I am still a strong and beautiful woman every damn day. It could be easier. The period is powerful. It is a bond between body and mind. A bond I intend to foster again.

Rain pours from the dark clouds above. I become saturated in cool and salty waters. I close my eyes, open my mouth, let it pour inside of me."

—Margaret Thompson, former client and amazing woman

If you are struggling with the symptoms of RED-S, please go to your primary care provider and get a checkup. Explain what you are doing, including how much you eat and your exercise schedule. They may not get it, but advocate for yourself. Don't expect that your coach will notice if you are having problems.

Bone density, breaks, and fractures

Even without the mental piece of an eating disorder, athletes (or very active people) are at a high risk of RED-S. This can come from a true ED, lack of nutrition education, or lack of access to food. A 2012 study examining high school athletes found that 41.5 percent of female high school athletes in "aesthetic sports" claimed disordered eating practices, and "were eight times more likely to incur an injury than athletes in aesthetic sports who did not report disordered eating." It's time to take a break and eat!

Exercise should not be resumed until you've recovered and are eating enough (as determined by your dietitian). Athletes who exercised while undereating (even at a "normal" weight) were still doing damage to their bones and were more susceptible to fractures. Your body is telling you it is not "fixed" yet. You can only gain bone density (strength) until your mid-20s. After that, you are just working to minimize loss. Build it while you can and know that food is your medicine.

Fractures

"I stress fractured both of my femurs within six months of each other in 2016. I was never a person who had bone-related injuries until I came to college—but then again, I was never a person who starved herself until then either. What I didn't realize at the time was all of my worst injuries occurred after long periods of diet restriction and over-exercising.

If you're not a serious athlete, it's hard to convey what injuries feel like to us—devastating is the best word I can use. To have worked so hard in training all summer and suffer a season-ending injury before you even get a chance to compete. Fast forward to admitting I had an ED and finally being in recovery, and realizing all those injuries were completely avoidable.

How many more times are you willing to go through that process? Asking for help and learning to be healthy/sustainable in both my diet and my life is how I went the longest periods without injury and ran my fastest times. No, the process is not going to be easy, but it will be worth it."

—Jessica Cushing-Murray

Athletes

Don't be afraid to talk to your coach. They are generally more understanding than you may expect. If they've worked in their position for any length of time, they have seen eating disorders and excessive exercise before. In fact, studies explained that 91 percent of athletic trainers have dealt with athletes with eating disorders, and 93 percent said there should be more attention paid to eating issues among their athletes. The downside is that only 27 percent of athletic trainers in college settings felt they could confidently identify disordered eating among their athletes. What's more, 25 percent of the colleges that were studied did not have a policy for management of eating disorders.

I won't bore you with more statistics (www. nationaleatingdisorders.org has a lot of them), but know that athletes of all ages, and especially those in weight class and aesthetic sports are at increased risk of disordered eating and eating disorders. If you are a struggling athlete, talk to your coach or trainer, see if your school has a counseling center or eating disorder specialists on-site, and ask for referrals to experts who can help you. Try to find a registered dietitian who specializes in sports nutrition and eating disorders, as they can help you discover the appropriate amounts of nutrients needed to fuel your body, leading to better performance and bone density.

Comparison is the thief of joy and self-identity

"Comparison was one of the bigger monsters I had to tackle in my eating disorder. It was how my ED started—I got to college and realized that many of my distance runner teammates were very thin and some didn't seem to eat very much.

I wrote in my journal from my time at UCLA: "All I know is that there are a lot of things a 19-year-old college sophomore could wish for…but all I want is to be skinny." I wanted the skinny

---

> *legs of one teammate and the bony arms/shoulders of another. I wanted basically any of their bodies—as long as it would get me out of my own.*
>
> *But continually comparing myself to my teammates was time-consuming, painful, and only exacerbated the problem I had. What made me feel better was recovery. What made me feel better was finally seeking help for the problem I had been struggling through on my own for years. What made me feel better was when I began to truly realize and understand that **my body is my own, and I don't need to look like anyone else to accomplish my goals and live my best life.** Always remember: you can't hate yourself into a version of yourself you can love."*
>
> —Jessica Cushing-Murray

So you need to limit your exercise

This can be one of the hardest things if you have been struggling with compulsive exercise. If your health-care providers are telling you to limit your exercise or are giving you specific recommendations for what you are allowed to do, realize we do not do this lightly. We know you won't want to follow it, and it is far less stressful to give you easier goals, but we ask you to cut back (or stop) exercising because we are worried about your health.

Your dietitian and health-care provider will give you specific restrictions based on your individual needs. Some general rules are:

- Weight should be maintained for about a month before increasing exercise amounts.
- As exercise increases, food intake will likely need to increase as well. Make sure you are mentally prepared for this.
- If your heart rate or blood pressure (or EKG) is not where it should be, then exercise really needs to be medically monitored! Cardiac arrest is never worth a workout.
- Noncompliance with a meal plan your RD gives you is a reason to limit exercise further.
- A minimum of one to two rest days per week is good for everyone. If you are dealing with an ED or over-exercise, this likely needs to increase to several rest days per week.

If you are on a team, you may be asked to take a leave from your sport. Your health MUST come before your sport. Appointments with your providers should not be skipped to practice or compete. Again, we are not doing this to punish you, but rather to ensure your safety and the longevity of your athletic career. It's far better to take a semester off than to push through and have serious complications like heart issues, fractures that will set you back a heck of a lot longer, or even death.

To help, put some barriers in your way. Make it hard to get to your athletic shoes and gear or give it to someone not in your home. Cancel your gym membership. Make other plans that do not involve much movement (like movie nights with friends). What are the things you've been missing out on because of "having to" exercise? Make time for them.

Finding joyful movement—what is appropriate exercise?

Exercise and activity should (I hate using the word "should," but it fits here) be something you enjoy, not a punishment! There are so many ways to move your body that you can find something different for every day of the year. What types of movement bring you joy?

Humans are meant to be in motion, as in we are not meant to be sedentary; but we are not built to go full-out for hours every day either. Assuming you are cleared to exercise, ask yourself "what actually feels good in my body today?" It can (and will) change daily. Some days, you will want complete rest or maybe gentle movement like yoga. Other days, you will have boundless energy and want to run, climb, and leap. On other days still, you'll feel like hitting or moving heavy things. It's all good, and good to change it up.

The thing to remember is why are you doing this? Because it feels good? Or because you feel obligated? Listen to your body!

Main takeaways:

- Nutrition varies for different types of activity, and as you increase movement, food intake needs to increase.
- Relative Energy Deficiency in Sport may not include the mental disorder of an ED, but it is still very serious! Pay attention to your needs and exercise amounts.
- Exercise restriction is done for your safety, not as a punishment.

- Move in ways that feel good—and rest is okay!

Take action:

If you are struggling to know what or how much to eat for your sport or activity, please seek a RD who specializes in sport nutrition.

If you are struggling with an ED or not knowing how to take care of your body, please talk to your athletic trainer or coach, and seek a therapist who specializes in ED. They can't help if they don't know what is going on.

Make sure you are taking rest days!

What is your resting heart rate? Check it for a few days. If it is low, get to a doctor or hospital ASAP!

Take a few minutes a day to stretch and practice your balance. One thing to try (if you are feeling steady enough) is balancing on one foot while you brush your teeth.

Chapter 7

Deal With It: Better Ways To Cope

"If hunger isn't the problem, food isn't the solution."

—Anonymous

The ED mindset grows in difficult times because eating disorders are a way of coping with emotions. In fact, it's very rarely about food or weight. Eating behaviors are a way to try and regulate emotions and "control" your environment when other things seem out of control. Transitions in life or stressful events create the potential for big emotional shifts that we might subconsciously try to dampen or numb. This can cause disordered eating behaviors and thoughts to pop up.

There are a lot of different ways to cope in stressful situations, and you don't have to pick just one! Different types of skills can be used in different situations. Let's start with what, in my opinion, is the most important: crisis plans.

Crisis plans

Do you have trustworthy people who you can talk to when you feel particularly stressed out? Or when you feel like you're going to binge, purge, have suicidal thoughts, or any other emotional reactions? Maybe a friend or family member, or your therapist, dietitian, doctor, mentor, or a crisis hotline?

Do you have any of those people saved in your phone or front of mind when a triggering situation comes up? Really think about it. When was the last time you leaned on someone for support instead of engaging in ED behaviors? If you said, "every time I think about doing [ED behavior], I instead talk to [specific person] and the desire goes away," then disregard this section (and WAY TO GO!).

If you didn't, then I want you to take out a small piece of paper that will fit in your wallet or create a note in your phone. Write down at least three people or hotlines you can call (or physically visit) in an emergency. This can be your therapist (only if they take emergency calls), a friend or family member who is helpful to your recovery (not someone who doesn't get it or will tear you down), or whoever can talk you down from your usual or most dangerous thoughts and behaviors. I also want you to list local police and suicide or crisis hotline numbers depending on your needs.

HOTLINES

In the US, the National Eating Disorders Association has a helpline: (800) 931-2237. Check the website for their hours of availability, as they aren't available 24 hours a day (currently, at the time of writing, the hours are M–Th: 9AM to 9PM EST, and 9–5 EST on Fridays).

NEDA also has a text crisis line. Individuals in the US can text "NEDA" to 741741 to connect with a crisis counselor 24/7.

Additionally, NEDA has an online chat function at: https://www.nationaleatingdisorders.org/help-support/ contact-helpline

National (US) suicide hotline (available 24 hours every day): 1-800-273-8255
TTY - Hearing & Speech Impaired: 1-800-799-4TTY

A crisis/suicide hotline for LGBTQ and youth, the Trevor Project, is a 24/7 phone crisis line. Call 1-866-488-7386. There is also an online chat available select hours at: https://www.thetrevorproject.org/.

Put these numbers in your wallet, purse, backpack, and phone so you have them with you all the time. If you've thought of these things ahead of time, you're more likely to reach out and get help. And if you get help, you're less likely to do dangerous things....Oh, and most importantly, USE IT WHEN YOU

NEED TO! These people are of no use if you don't contact them when you need help. *There is no shame in asking for help.*

Sexual assault

Unfortunately, many eating disorders persist because of trauma like sexual assault or rape. Many women (and increasingly other genders) who were raped or molested at a young age use food not only as a way to numb themselves from having to think about it, but as a protective shield used for trying to be less desirable (extra weight), trying to be invisible (underweight/not go out), or hiding their mature ("sexy") curves. This is deep trauma that can be held in the subconscious. A lot of my clients never even realized they were using food. It can also turn into a form of substance abuse that leads to "checking out" and not being "present" in life.

Delaying behaviors

Delaying ED behaviors is a great way to slowly work yourself out of an ED. I mentioned this in chapter 5 "how to stop purging." For this section, I'm going to use the example of binge eating, but you can apply your specific behaviors in its place. It's important to realize that the action often becomes mindless. If we do something consistently, a habit develops. We don't realize that we're in a binge until we're halfway through it or done with it. Therefore, I want you to start bringing awareness when you're going into a binge. Try to look at your food journal to help figure out triggers, or to bring more awareness to yourself when you're feeling that need to binge. Once you've figured out that a binge is about to happen, I want you to work on delaying the binge. I'm not saying that it doesn't have to happen. Ideally, down the road, we'll get to not needing to binge, but for right now just focus on delaying it for at least 20 minutes.

For those 20 minutes, utilize a distracting coping method such as going for a walk, talking to a friend, creating art, or even drinking a glass of water. Feel free to use any healthy self-care or behavior tips on the list below. Hopefully, in that 20 or more minutes, you will become engrossed in your distraction and eventually learn to delay the behavior for hours.

A couple of things will happen in the process. One, an immediate urge to binge will go away, therefore you won't *need* to binge, even though it may still happen. And for right now, that's okay. You will become more aware of your emotional triggers and lose that impulsivity in the future. The longer we can continue to delay a binge, the better. Maybe today, you make it 10 minutes. Great! That's 10 minutes longer than you've had before. Maybe, a week from now, you're delaying it to 20 to 30 minutes. Soon, you're delaying for several hours. Eventually, you won't need to do it at all. This is breaking a habit, people!

It's okay that these urges come up. Urges happen. We will feel an urge to binge, to restrict, to purge, to [insert behavior]. It's our reactions to those urges that we can change. By delaying, we are still feeling what's happening and acting to postpone the behavior. Continue to build on this foundation until you don't need to use your ED behavior anymore.

There is hope for full recovery

"I believe that full recovery is possible, and the difficult journey to get there is worth it, because I am living proof from both a personal and professional perspective! My own recovery story overlapped my first few years as a clinical dietitian working at a hospital—proof that knowledge is not the answer to healing.

Recovery takes honesty, vulnerability, and faith in your treatment team to hold hope for you until you can hold it on your own. I am so grateful for those who believed in me and taught me how to believe in myself and my recovery. Recovery gave me back my own life and opened the door to a career that I am as passionate about today as I was that first time I sat across from my first client as a newly recovered dietitian who couldn't wait to help someone find hope again."

—Tammy Beasley, RDN, CEDRD, CSSD, LD
Vice President of Clinical Nutrition Services for Alsana (a well-known treatment center)

What's eating you?

Once you have several days or weeks of recording in your food journal (from chapter 2) and identifying barriers and triggers in your eating patterns, you can begin to look at other barriers and triggers in your life. These are things that are either going to help or hinder your recovery, both from your eating disorder and from other difficulties or challenges.

We need to look at the bigger picture; what is your lifestyle like? Don't just look at your mealtimes, but also consider the people that you are hanging out with. Are they supportive of your recovery or are they enabling you to continue these behaviors? It is said that you are the sum of the five people you spend the most time with. Who do you want to be? It is important to spend more time around people who are going to lift you up and help you move forward, whether this is in terms of recovery or any other part of your life.

Additionally, look at the actual food around you, not just the food environment. What foods do you keep in your house? Do you have easy access to a grocery store? Are you shopping with a list to make sure you're getting ingredients to actually make meals, or are you just impulse-buying snack foods and never cooking full meals (or getting too overwhelmed to buy any food)? Do you eat out all the time and feel unsure about how to create meals on your own? Are you facing food insecurity (not enough money or access to food)? Take a step back and ask yourself, "Where are my problem areas?"

What positive changes do you need to make? Do you need to take a cooking class or look up recipes? Shop with a grocery list? Visit a food pantry or apply for financial assistance or SNAP benefits ("food stamps")?

Back to the food journal. Go through it and see your most difficult days and the corresponding triggers (this is where keeping detailed info on who/where/thoughts is helpful). If you're having days when you're hardly eating because you're spending time around people who make you feel bad about yourself, know that not eating will not fix the problem! Alternatively, if you're having days when you spent time around people who make you feel awful about yourself, only to go home, eat a family-size bag of Doritos and a pint of ice cream in your room, it may be time to take a step back. It's not just the fact that that food was there. Whether that food was in your house, or you bought it on the way home, there's always a way to access food, so look deeper. How did you feel around those people? What could you have done instead?

People in our lives are going to say dumb and rude things. We can't control other people. If someone gives you a negative comment and you internalize it, instead of automatically reaching for the food or believing that taking control of your food and weight will make you feel better, take a moment and ask yourself a few questions: "What did they say? How am I feeling about that? Is that something that's actually true or is it their issue?"

Most of the time, the things people say are not about us. It's about them. Humans are very egocentric, especially in their teen years (before the brain has fully developed, around age 25). Everyone has their own blinders that keep them focused on "me, me, me." Putting others down is usually based on their own insecurity. For example, if someone calls you "fat," it is not about you. It is their own fear of becoming "fat," or their need to assert power over you. It doesn't mean it is true.

Most things said maliciously aren't coming from a place of truth. Often, the person is really hurting and taking anger out on you. If you're feeling comfortable, you could always talk to them about it. If not, chalk it up to experience and remind yourself that food or exercise isn't going to change their behavior or make you feel better.

We can apply this to other situations as well. I know comments often trigger us, but there are many other types of triggers. It could be a book or a movie that set off an emotional trigger. It could also be a situation such as a social gathering that generates anxiety. You may find yourself leaning on food instead of enjoying the company. Or maybe, it stresses you out so much that you go home and binge or skip eating altogether.

Look at those scenarios and think about whether or not food is really the answer. I promise you, it's really not. Try finding an action that will actually improve these scenarios. If it's social anxiety, for instance, perhaps spend more time in therapy and say no to some events. Maybe you do need to go to your best friend's birthday party, but not to a networking event or club meeting. Choosing the scenarios you are going to engage allows you to limit the number of triggering situations until you have fully worked through your anxiety.

Therapy

Many people have different coping mechanisms that are not healthy. Some people drink too much, gamble, or abuse drugs as ways to cope. These addictions also place them at higher risk of flip-flopping back and forth with eating disorder behaviors if underlying needs are not met because they all serve the same purpose of numbing or creating a "high." For the immediate future, we're going to be looking at better ways to cope. In the long term, I want you to work on solving the root of the problem. This is typically where psychotherapy comes in handy.

Sorry, Freud, it's not all about you

I love therapy. It's a place where I can be completely me without feeling judged. Instead, I feel listened to and helped to be my best self. Once a big stigma, therapy has become widely accepted in many cultures. Everyone can benefit from some form of therapy, as we all have our "stuff." Now there are many treatment modalities to choose from, so find a good fit for you. It's not all Freudian anymore.

It may be a past trauma that you need to fully process before moving on. Thankfully, there are many therapists who have been trained to work with trauma. If you're facing a current emotional or relational issue, it is important to learn how to navigate it. What will help you recover from your ED is action that allows you to address the emotional problem. Until you can get a grasp on the underlying *why*, it may be very difficult to let go of ED behaviors and be truly free.

There are different ways to cope that are healthier for your body and mind than eating disorder behaviors or substance abuse. Below is a list of different, healthier, coping skills that you can be using. This way you can have different types of coping skills that you enjoy and that work in different moments and situations in your life. I've broken these skills down into certain categories to help you if you feel really stuck.

★ Coping skills

Self-Soothing:

- Use your five senses: Find something pleasant to touch, taste, see, hear, and smell (this is also called a grounding technique). Take it up a notch by finding five things you can see, four things you can touch, three things you can hear, two things you can smell, and one thing you can taste.
- Body scan: Check in with your body, starting at your toes and working your way up. You can also do progressive muscle relaxation. Tense single body parts for a few seconds, then let them release along with the accumulated tension in that area as you move up the body.
- Go on a "social-media fast" by either logging off for a day, week, or month, or delete accounts entirely, (If you can't bring yourself to completely disengage, or have to use them for work like me, at least unfollow any accounts that make you feel bad about yourself.)

Distractions:

- Read a book
- Listen to music
- Knit/crochet/needlepoint
- Make art
- Do a puzzle (cardboard, word, number, whatever you like)
- Movie night with a friend
- Go for a walk
- Clean/declutter

- Adult coloring books (it's a thing)
- Learn something new (massive open online courses, book, community education)
- Paint your nails
- Play board games
- Play video games (something uplifting is best)
- Watch a TED Talk online
- Volunteer
- Watch funny videos on YouTube (SNL, anyone?)
- Write a letter (you definitely know someone who wants snail mail)
- Make fun plans for a trip or event

Physical:

- Joyful movement (skip, hike, fitness class, whatever—as long as it is not excessive)
- Yoga/stretching
- Eat a balanced meal (carbs, proteins, and fats)
- Dance
- Play with animals (walk a dog or help at a shelter if you don't have your own)
- Swim
- Get out in nature
- Go horseback riding
- Shoot hoops (basketball) or arrows (archery)
- Throw your shoes at a wall (make sure it won't be damaged; concrete is good for this)
- Take a bath
- Rearrange a room
- Try a new recipe you have been wanting to make

Opposite Action:

- Positive affirmations (find online, tell yourself in the mirror, read positive books)
- See/read something funny or happy (comedy show, funny movie, jokes)
- Gratitude journal/share something good or that you are proud of today
- Pay it forward: buy coffee (or something) for a stranger
- Take a shower and put on clean clothes that make you feel confident
- Write motivational quotes on Post-its and post around the house (or the community, to inspire others)
- Go socialize with friends/get out of the house

Emotional Awareness:

- Journal feelings
- Create art that lets your emotions out
- Go to a therapy session
- Talk to a friend you really trust
- Tell someone how much they mean to you
- Forgive someone
- Celebrate accomplishments!
- Avoid triggers (know yourself)
- Use "No" as a complete sentence and set boundaries
- Take a nap if you are tired
- Do not believe the things you tell yourself late at night

Mindfulness:

- Meditation or prayer
- Breathing exercises

- Mindful eating
- Use grounding objects (a "touchstone" to keep with you, like a small stone)
- Relaxation recordings to listen to (positive visualizations or led-meditations)
- Drink a glass of water or tea
- Turn your phone OFF
- Go outside and look at the details in the world
- Make a list of your accomplishments
- Create a vision board, Pinterest board, or goal list

Practical Self-Care:

- Make a grocery list, and have a set time to go every week
- Don't overspend/spend unwisely (set a budget and stick to it)
- Pick up things when you are done (don't leave things lying around)
- Declutter your space (clutter = chaos in the mind)
- Batch-cook and freeze meals in single servings
- Delete old emails and "unfriend" people who bring you down
- Keep your big "to-dos" to three or fewer per day
- Use a planner or calendar (you can't remember everything)
- Take one small step towards your bigger goal
- Wake up and go to bed at the same time every day

Have a Crisis Plan:

- Crisis phone #: _____
- Police phone #: _____
- Therapist/Psychiatrist:_____

- Friend(s) to call: _____

  _____

  _____

  _____

- Local Emergency Room: _____

  _____

Avoiding lapses and relapses

Something many people forget when they are in a good place with their ED recovery is that life transitions, even good ones, are potential triggers for behaviors or thoughts. Even when you are feeling recovered and strong, you need to keep a back-of-the-mind awareness of thoughts and behaviors that you thought were long gone. If you notice that your go-to coping skills are ED behaviors, please act early! You know the hell you went through before. Do you want that again?

Relapses and lapses (a "slip-up" rather than a complete relapse) are always a risk, even when recovery is going really well. Unless better coping skills have been practiced and made new habits, ED behaviors often return when stress or transitions inevitably show up again.

Quick tip if you are someone who "forgets" to eat: Set alarms on your cell phone to remind you to stop and eat something. Packing food with you, meal prepping, and always having ingredients for go-to meals can also help.

Good times and bad

I think one of the hardest parts of working through your ED is staying motivated when you are having a bad day, which will happen.

Try this: when you are having a good day (especially a good body image day), write down what that feels like. Be very specific. Why do you feel good? What does it mean to not care about what you look like or believe you are fabulous as you are? When you have energy from eating more, write down how good that makes you feel and what a difference eating makes. Then, when you are having a rough day, re-read what you wrote. The fact that the words came from you—that you spoke your own truth and that you actually felt good—will help you push through on the hard days.

Main takeaways:

- There is no shame in asking for help.
- There are lots of different coping skills that you can use in place of self-regulating with food or exercise. Try a variety of them and make sure to have a crisis plan in place.
- EDs can flip-flop with other addictions if underlying issues are not addressed and better coping skills are not developed into go-to habits.
- Lapses will happen. Practice good coping skills now to make sure they don't turn into full relapses later.

Take action (grab your journal):

Pull out your journal and take a few minutes to think about why you use food and/or exercise as your way of avoiding things. More importantly, identify what you are avoiding.

Delay an ED behavior for 20 minutes next time the urge comes up. Have some potential distractions that you can use from the coping skills list (or your own ideas). How did it go? Did the urge decrease? Keep delaying until you can go for a long time, eventually rendering the behavior useless.

Take a few minutes and write down the barriers in your life as well as the things or people who trigger you to reach for food. Also, be sure to note the things you can tell yourself in the moment to slow down. What I mean is that you will not jump from point A, which is a triggering behavior like someone's comment to you, to C, which is grabbing or avoiding food as a coping mechanism. I want you to focus on point B. What happens between A and C? Ultimately, you can't control the events that are triggering you, but you can control what happens in the interim. When you make this effort, you can stop the tendency to use food as a behavioral coping mechanism.

When you are having a good day (especially a good body image day), write down what that feels like. Be very specific. Why do you feel good?

Pick a few coping skills from the list and make sure to have any supplies easily accessible. For example: if you want to color, have markers or pencils and paper or a coloring book together and near where you like to sit or pass by frequently.

Chapter 8

Doctors, Dietitians, and Therapists, Oh My!

"If you talk about it, it's a dream. If you envision it, it's possible. But if you schedule it, it's real."

—Tony Robbins

When struggling with eating, whether or not you are ready to recover, whether it has been 1 month or 20 years, you really need to be honest with your health-care providers about what is going on.

I have had several clients who were not honest about their ED behaviors with me or another health-care provider and it really delayed their treatment and recovery, sometimes in devastating ways. I don't want that to happen to you. I hope that I can help you feel more comfortable about the information you should share and trust that we are here to help you, not judge you.

Why is it so important to tell your health-care providers about your eating behaviors? Shouldn't they be able to tell if something is wrong?

I mean, that would be amazing, but eating disorders are sneaky! For one, usually, they look "normal" in terms of weight, blood tests, and more, until it is late in the disease process. Additionally, many providers are still under the impression that someone has to be emaciated to have an eating disorder, which is of course not true! You can't tell if someone has issues with food or body image just by looking at them (more on this in chapter 9).

The average doctor's visit is under 15 minutes. In that time, they need to assess every part of you, and if you don't speak up and say what is wrong they might not catch a problem or may gloss over it. They also do not have time to educate, dig deep into mental status, or follow up on referrals to see if you actually followed through. If you have longer visits, you are among the lucky. Take advantage of that time!

Getting medical checkups is absolutely essential. However, you might hear that you are "fine," "healthy," "at a normal weight," "overweight," or "you must be athletic because your heart rate is so low." These are not helpful statements for someone struggling with disordered eating or body image issues.

Doctors don't always "get it"

Some things medical providers said that did not help the situation:

"You're a nutrition major? Are you eating enough calcium?"
—My doctor at an appointment during my most restrictive phase of eating. She said I was fine. I was not okay, but I didn't know I had a problem.

"I prefer my patients to be underweight anyway. I wouldn't try to gain weight."
—A medical provider to Sarah Chapin when she was dealing with digestive issues in refeeding because of anorexia nervosa.

"With your knowledge, you should know not to engage in 'those' behaviors."
—A medical provider to their patient, a psychologist, when she was relapsing in her ED.

"Obviously, if you don't slow down [the weight gain/eating] you will end up obese."
—A doctor to Kat Furman at a routine weighing during recovery.
(For the record, becoming "obese" is not a big risk for those who struggled with anorexia. It can happen, but not typically.)

If eating disorders are disregarded, recovery can be difficult if not impossible. Additionally, medical conditions that are not externally visible can be doing major damage under the surface, as in the case of organ failure from malnutrition.

Who do you need to tell, and what do you need to tell them? Tell anyone who is involved in your health care, physical or mental. This includes but is not limited to: doctors, nurses, nurse practitioners, physician assistants, dietitians or nutritionists, therapists, massage therapists, psychiatrists, pharmacists, dermatologists, dentists (especially if purging), acupuncturists, midwives, fitness trainers (if you collapse, they need to know why), chiropractors, and anyone else who has an impact on your physical and mental health.

Not all of these people can do much about your eating disorder, nor are they all essential, but if you are only working with a massage therapist, for instance, they might be able to make a referral to a specialist that you otherwise wouldn't know about. A personal trainer needs to know what's going on, so they don't push a "visibly healthy" person to cardiac arrest with strenuous exercise.

You don't have to give the same amount of information to each of these people, but all of them should know the basics about what you're doing. Are you restricting your intake, fasting, or purging? How much are you exercising? Have you ever fainted or had other scary consequences from your eating disorder?

More information on the specifics should be given to your health-care providers (whether at a routine physical or in the hospital), your dietitian, therapist, psychiatrist, and anyone else you feel needs to know, or you feel comfortable telling. If we don't know what is actually going on, we may give suggestions or treatment that at best are not effective, at worst—deadly.

We work in health care because we want to help people get better, not worse. Don't be afraid to bring anything up with us. We are not here to judge, and believe me, we have heard it all, especially the longer we have been in practice. You might think something you do, or a symptom you experience, is not relevant, but bring it up anyway—you never know what we might be looking for. We don't always have right the questions. You're not blabbering, I want to hear your story.

Another upside to telling your providers is that you can ask to not be weighed. You can also ask for "blind weights," where you do not see the number and they don't talk about your weight.

If you don't have an eating disorder specialist yet, your initial contact can make referrals or point you in the right direction so you get the best care in a setting that works for you. This is important because many health-care providers do not have a lot of training in eating disorders and may not have the latest information on treatment or know how to speak in non-triggering ways. If you do not feel your provider understands the disorder, you have every right to ask for second and third opinions. You know your body best, but ED lies; so make sure you are not shying away from objective opinions either.

Live the life you want right now.

Not when you lose the weight.
Not when you finish the degree.
Not when you get the job/partner/accolade/kid/kid moves out.
You are worthy just as you are. Live life right now.

Specifically, who should you have on your recovery team? In the clinical world, this is called an "interdisciplinary treatment team" of professionals who (ideally) talk to each other to make sure everyone is on the same page about your individualized needs. They should be experienced in successfully working with EDs.

At a bare minimum, a physician (MD, PA, or NP) should be monitoring if you are medically stable and checking vital signs, labs, and other markers of physical and mental health. If possible, look for the initials "CEDS" after their name. This is "Certified Eating Disorder Specialist." There are not many relative to the number of physicians out there, so it's not a deal breaker.

Next, you will want to find a Registered Dietitian (RD or RDN) to help you with the food piece. RDs are legally credentialed to provide "medical nutrition therapy" that "nutritionists" cannot.

"All Registered Dietitians are Nutritionists, but not all Nutritionists are Registered Dietitians"

— Academy of Nutrition and Dietetics

Ideally, a CEDRD, or "Certified Eating Disorder Registered Dietitian," or an RD who has lots of experience with EDs should be sought out. If any professional puts you on a diet or says to not eat certain foods or food groups, find someone else. RDs help people figure out what and how much to eat, how to overcome barriers to eating, how to develop a good relationship with food and your body, and how to make behavioral changes. A good RD will look at your whole lifestyle, not just food, including your emotional needs, living situation, food preferences, activity levels, and more. We don't eat just based on nutrient needs, and therefore generic meal plans are not the best bet.

Do you have trouble following your treatment plan?

I've included some brilliant insights from participants in a recovery group I recently led. They shed light on why it can be so hard to follow a treatment plan, even when you know it's good for you.

ED is often an outlet for anger or desire for attention. And when the ED voice is loud, you probably feel like you are a failure if you do the ED behaviors, and a failure if you don't do the ED behaviors. For those of you that feel a rebellious streak, think about being defiant or rebelling against ED, rather than "pleasing" or "obeying" your treatment team.

Channel anger against ED (who doesn't have a face) instead of people (who do have a face).
Say, "f*ck you, ED!"
Be defiant!

A psychotherapist is another must on the team. Depending on where you live, they have different titles such as "licensed marriage family therapist" (LMFT), "licensed professional clinical counselor" (LPCC), "psychologist" (PsyD), "licensed clinical social worker" (LCSW), or others. Again, look for ED experience. If possible, a "CEDS" is ideal. Find someone with whom you feel comfortable. A good therapist will use different techniques to help you work through mental needs.

An optional addition to your team may be a recovery coach or a support group. These can be a big help to keep you accountable between sessions with your other professionals, but shouldn't be the only resources you employ, as they cannot tackle your specific medical, dietary, or complex mental health needs.

Lastly, a psychiatrist may be needed as indicated by your other professionals. Psychiatrists are mainly for medication management and mental assessment, especially if you are dealing with other mental illness along with the ED. Look for someone with ED experience. Hopefully, your other professionals can make referrals.

Check Appendix A for places to look for professionals in your area and first steps to getting professional help if you are stuck.

Tracking apps

Do you track your food on an app? Tracking what you eat is a common practice in weight management, and with the rise of technology there are hundreds of apps to use if you don't like pen and paper. I know apps like "My Fitness Pal," and trackers like "Fitbit," are super popular right now, not only among the fitness set, but among dieters and people using it to fuel their ED. These apps are not necessarily giving correct calorie goals and fuel the obsession with numbers.

This gives the impression that weight is something that we must control, no matter the cost. While there are benefits for some (making sure athletes are replacing glycogen stores, checking for nutrient deficiencies), for the general population

---

it is really not necessary (and very triggering for those with EDs!). In general, I do not recommend tracking apps. Eating is pretty simple if you can listen to your body and eat a variety of foods.

One app I do like (I have no affiliation with them) is "Recovery Record," which is a food, mood, and behavior tracker that you can link with your dietitian. It allows them to see what you eat in real time as you log, and it does not track calories. You can write descriptions of what you ate or take photos, list how you are feeling, your hunger levels, ED behaviors (such as body-checking or purging), and write secure messages back and forth with your treatment team. It is free for clients and low cost for providers.

★ How to talk to professionals when you are scared to see them

Are you scared to seek professional help? It's okay, we don't bite! The reason we get into this field is because we want to help you. If you are going to an ED specialist, there is a good chance we have struggled on some level with the same things and understand where you are coming from. While we can't get accurate statistics on this, several studies (and personal accounts from professionals) show that many eating disorder professionals have struggled with disordered eating themselves (just make sure you get the vibe that they are fully recovered before you work intensely with them).

When you go to your appointment, I suggest bringing a list of concerns and your food behaviors. Are you anxious? Chest pain? Vomiting? How much do you eat? Do you count calories/ otherwise track? What is your exercise regimen? It can help to write this down. If you are too nervous to talk about it, you can always hand them the list you made.

Once you meet, the therapist or dietitian can tell you more about what's going on in your body and give treatment recommendations (how often you need to meet, etc.). This really varies from person to person, from occasional check-ins, to weekly, to higher levels of care (up to 24 hours/day).

Remember, the food and exercise behaviors are just a coping mechanism for something deeper. You don't have to stay stuck in the cycle of damaging your body to avoid something. Recovery is hard to go alone. It's okay to get help.

Main takeaways:

- Recovery is a team approach. You need professionals with experience in eating disorders, and they should be communicating with each other to give you the best possible treatment.
- There is no need to track calories, macros, or exercise. Let it go.

Take action:

You have to take charge of your own health care. Find a provider. Make a list of concerns and behaviors to talk about when you get there, and if you can, give them a heads-up about the reason for the appointment. This will go far to ensure you get the best possible treatment.

If you have calorie tracking apps, delete them! If you feel a need to track in some way, try Recovery Record or ask your providers for recommended apps that don't revolve around calories and weight.

Chapter 9

But My Doctor Said I Look Perfect

"To live is the rarest thing in the world. Most people just exist."

—Oscar Wilde

Your doctor said everything looked perfect!

So what?

You can't rely on a quick doctor's visit to tell you if you have a problem with your eating. Very rarely are there objective, visible signs of an eating disorder. The fact that there aren't readily visible signs does not mean you are not struggling or that you are not doing harm to your body and mind.

Up until now, we've been focusing on the day-to-day stuff with ED, but I have to remind you that eating disorders are serious medical diseases in addition to mental illnesses and that anorexia nervosa has the highest rate of mortality (death) of *any* psychiatric illness (10 percent; 20 percent of those are by suicide, the majority of the other 80 percent are the result of heart failure)! Medical complications can sneak up on you. Pay attention!

In my practice, I have seen hundreds of people with eating disorders and looked at a whole lot of lab numbers. Most of those labs looked absolutely perfect, but that's not the whole picture.

For example, a client of mine had been taking ridiculous amounts of laxatives almost every day for months in addition to restricting, and her labs looked great. She was on the slim side of "normal weight." If her labs were the only information you got about her, you would think nothing was wrong, despite her having been stuck in the depths of a serious eating disorder for about 10 years!

Most people walking around with EDs have perfect blood work, are at "normal" or "healthy" weight (I hate using these terms, but that's society for you), and are at war with the ED voice in their head all day long.

EDs are an invisible disease for most. Because of the ever-present diet culture, you may be praised for losing weight, even if it's done in a very unhealthy way like restriction. While being asked, "Did you lose weight? You look great!" seems like a positive thing, it is one of the cultural norms that prevents us from fully trusting our bodies.

Despite the fact that labs rarely show issues, we want to be checking them on a regular basis to see if things are going downhill. Some problems can be fixed easily, while others necessitate a major intervention. Let's go over some of the common labs we want to be checking and what tends to show up first as red flags.

Labs typically ordered:

Complete blood count (CBC), comprehensive metabolic panel (CMP), thyroid, magnesium, phosphorus, vitamin D, potentially vitamin B12, urinalysis (specific gravity), orthostatic vitals (blood pressure and heart rate), and EKG (electrocardiogram) to check your heart.

Typical first lab issues I have seen are:

White blood cell counts (WBC) and liver function tests (AST and ALT) are some of the first labs that highlight problems related to considerable weight loss or restriction. Since all blood is filtered through our liver, this is an organ that can tell us the health of our blood pretty quickly.

Oddly enough, cholesterol may be high (hypercholesterolemia) in anorexia. Like most of the other labs, this tends to return to normal when the person eats enough on a regular basis. Watch carefully for hypoglycemia (low blood sugar) when restricting. This is a bigger deal than most people know and can cause a quick decline (even death).

In those who purge using vomiting or laxatives, serum bicarbonate can get thrown out of balance as the body struggles to maintain the correct pH (acid-base balance) in the blood and body fluids. This is NOT fixed by an "alkaline diet;" it is fixed by not purging. Not to mention the damage that stomach acid can do on the esophagus and mouth from vomiting.

Other issues with purging include decreased serum potassium, sodium, and magnesium. Along with calcium, these are your blood electrolytes. When low, they not only make you feel lethargic but can also stop your heart! An effort should be made to slowly increase your intake of them.

Another strange occurrence with repeated vomiting is something often referred to as "chipmunk cheeks," the swelling that you see in the lower parts of the jaw. This is parotid gland swelling from that acid coming up. It will go away after vomiting stops for a while.

In addition to blood work, it is important to have your vital signs checked—resting heart rate and blood pressure. These should be checked from lying down to standing. A big drop in blood pressure with a big rise in heart rate is called orthostatic hypotension, and it is caused by your body not being able to maintain blood around your brain (which is necessary) at the normal rate. This causes you to feel dizzy or faint when you stand up.

Heart rate is often an early indicator of issues related to anorexia specifically. As the body is undernourished, heart rate slows down to conserve energy—your heart literally can't spare an extra beat as there is not enough energy from calories. Resting heart rates under 50 beats per minute should be looked at by a trained medical professional. For anything under 40, go to urgent care or the emergency room!

Perfectionism & straight As

Kaylie* is a straight-A, pre-med student. Her time is spent studying, volunteering, applying to internships, and running. She is on track to graduate a year early and go to medical school to be a dermatologist or pediatrician. What you wouldn't know if you meet her is that she has a horrible relationship with food, and over the past year she has not gotten her period, has lost weight, and a recent scan showed her bone density is much lower than it should be for a 19-year-old.

Under all the report cards, this bright student is a quivering ball of anxiety. She feels pressure not only from her parents, but also herself to get into med school. She's not even sure she wants to be a doctor, but it sounds like a great job and she wants to help people.

In high school, she ran track and cross country, and she made the team going into her first year at college. Running every day while trying to keep up with hard classes made Kaylie feel overwhelmed. She was so tired, her run times were getting slower. Noticing that many of the other girls on the team were very thin, she assumed she was slower because she wasn't "as thin" as they were. Losing weight means cutting time, right?

One day, Kaylie decides she is no longer going to snack. She reads some blog posts about nutrition and makes herself a meal plan that looks very healthy. She starts to lose weight. It's working!

The problem is that she gets so hungry at the end of the day that a few days a week, she finds herself on the other side of a binge—eating her roommate's food! She feels discouraged. The perfectionist can't hold herself to a "healthy" eating plan. Where is her willpower?

I meet Kaylie at this point. She has been referred to me by a therapist who she saw for feeling discouraged and depressed. After talking with her, I find out she is feeling out of control. She finds school hard, and is not excited about becoming a doctor, but hasn't felt able to bring it up with her parents because that is all that they talk about. Running isn't that fun anymore. It is a lot of work running when she is exhausted, and she compares herself to every girl on the team, convinced they are all thinner, fitter, faster, and have better willpower than her. And she feels ashamed that she can't eat without binging. In reality, she has not eaten enough calories to sustain her body for months. She is depressed, anxious, and in a spiral of binging, purging, and restricting.

I wish I could say this was a unique scenario.

Restrictive eating disorders and perfectionism go together like peanut butter and jelly. There are personality traits I, and other professionals, have noted as matching each ED. With restriction in any form, and often bulimia, there is a big push towards perfectionism and when we look at what is going wrong in a person's life and health, grades are often the last thing to slip.

*name changed (and she is doing really well now)

Food makes you happy in more ways than one

"You are what you eat" extends to mental health. Neurotransmitters (brain chemicals like serotonin and dopamine) are completely dependent upon our diet for synthesis. Carbohydrates and certain amino acids in food (like tyrosine) are needed to make our neurotransmitters. When you are not eating enough, lacking variety, or purging out food needed to make them, these chemicals cannot be made. What does it matter?

Well, our brain chemicals are responsible for staving off depression and anxiety! Serotonin is our "happy" neurochemical. When it is lacking or out of balance, we experience depression. Dopamine is our "pleasure" neurochemical. It creates the "high" feelings from fun things like winning a game. The other major brain chemical related to EDs is norepinephrine, our "adrenaline" neurotransmitter (as well as hormone). This creates the fight-or-flight response.

If we do not have enough of these neurotransmitters being made by the body (from lack of food), then we experience depression, anxiety, and other mental illness. This appears to be why anxiety and depression are so common in people with EDs. There is no literature supporting the use of selective serotonin reuptake inhibitors, SSRIs (a class of antidepressant medication that works on serotonin), for anorexia. This research goes back to the work of Ancel Keys in the 1940s with a starvation experiment in which he realized that, unless carbohydrate intake was sufficient, SSRIs did not work. I'm no psychiatrist, but that makes sense given how the neurotransmitters are made in the body.

Antidepressant medications (SSRIs and SNRIs) are selective serotonin/norepinephrine reuptake inhibitors, which means they prevent serotonin or norepinephrine from being taken back up into their storage sites and thus allows them to be used as intended by the brain. If there is not enough serotonin or other neurochemicals, however, it doesn't matter if the medications are taken; they're not going to be effective. Additionally, there is newer research showing that there are genetic predispositions that can make you more resistant to certain medications. In other words, even the maximum dose won't have a great effect on you because the blood levels required by the medication cannot build up enough.

So, what do we do? The medication for EDs that has to be taken FIRST is FOOD. Without enough food, nothing gets better. Then, cognitive behavioral therapy (CBT) for most people. This is still the "gold standard" of therapy for eating disorders. However, it's not the right fit for everyone, so be open to trying different types of therapy, like dialectical behavioral therapy (DBT), acceptance and commitment therapy (ACT), eye movement desensitization and reprocessing (EMDR), and others. Find a psychotherapist and registered dietitian you trust.

How do food and nutrients in particular really act as "medicine"? To be clear, I am not knocking real medications— take them when needed in conjunction with a balanced diet. Back to the question, there is a lot of evidence for medical nutrition therapy (what RDs do) for many diseases including mental health issues like depression and anxiety.

Research into nutrition for mental health is relatively new in the scheme of scientific research, but there are a lot of promising studies in the last five to ten years showing the impact of specific elements of food on the brain. We already discussed carbohydrates and amino acids for serotonin production, but other foods have had a significant impact on brain function as well. The first goal for nutrition therapy in EDs is to make sure you are getting an adequate number of calories. Then, balancing macronutrient levels and only thereafter specific nutrients, which can have a great impact on the brain as well as the body. A study from 2017 by Opie et al. stated, "Any protective effects are likely to come from the cumulative and synergic effect of nutrients that comprise the whole-diet, rather than from the effects of individual nutrients or single foods."

Starting with the broader diet, several studies have shown that dietary patterns like those in the Mediterranean, Norwegian, and Japanese cultures (specifically, lacto-pescatarian diets) are among the most preventative for depression and mood disorders, whereas the stereotypical Western American diet (specifically, the higher levels of saturated fats and added sugars) has been shown to increase the risk of depression in studies that followed participants for many years. As with all scientific studies, there is plenty of room for more research.

So, what do we do? Overall: eating enough, balancing the macros (carbs, proteins, fats), and eating more Mediterranean-style diet patterns. Once you're there, I have included a list of some of the more specific nutrients to focus on.

Omega-3 polyunsaturated fatty acids (n-3 PUFA), like those found in fish oil, flax seed, chia seeds, fatty fish, and walnuts, have been the focus of several studies on depression. One study specifically linked a lack of n-3 PUFAs in the diet with an increased likelihood of depression. Other studies looked at n-3 PUFA supplements and the reduction of depression. Still other studies that did not look at this nutrient specifically did say that dietary patterns (mentioned above) helped with depression, all of which are known for their higher than average levels of n-3 PUFAs. I'm sold!

Probiotics, the helpful bacteria we eat, and our overall gut microbiota, have had a lot of buzz around the way it decreases depression! Probiotics are found in fermented foods like yogurt, kefir, sauerkraut, kimchee, as well as supplements (often found in the refrigerated section). Pinto-Sanchez et al. studied the effects of one specific strain of probiotic bacteria, *Bifidobacterium longum NCC3001*. They found that this strain of bacteria created significant decreases in depression (though not anxiety) in people with IBS. This bacteria seemed to create changes in certain parts of the brain, especially those related to limbic reactivity. Look for this strain of bacteria in your yogurt or probiotic supplements.

B vitamins were mentioned in many studies as having a beneficial effect on mood disorders. Focus on whole grains, legumes, fruit (especially citrus), veggies, nuts, and seeds most of all. If you do not eat any animal products, add a B12 supplement (otherwise, B12 is found only in animal products and fortified nutritional yeast).

Hormones

Our body produces a lot of hormones made from proteins and fats, which can be lowered or made dysfunctional in an eating disorder. Here are a few that can become an issue.

Thyroid hormones (from the gland in your neck) might be abnormal (high or low) as a result of an eating disorder, especially anorexia. Our thyroid regulates energy, metabolism, temperature, menstruation, and more. The good news is that if the thyroid is off because of ED, it usually corrects itself with proper nutrition and rest. This is a good reason to step up the recovery process—a dysfunctional thyroid makes life miserable.

Continuing on the topic of amenorrhea from chapter 6, to get your period back and have healthy levels of hormones, proper nutrition and typically weight gain are necessary. Getting back to the weight you lost it at (plus perhaps an additional five pounds) usually results in your period returning. Hormone therapy or oral contraceptives should never be used to induce a period.

Young women are not the only ones at risk for hormonal problems. Older women who have hit menopause are still at risk of hormonal (and other) problems with their ED, and men of any age can have issues with testosterone levels. Especially in the teen and young adult years, males who are not eating enough can have low levels of testosterone, which can delay development (growth and sexual development), lower bone density, make it difficult to gain muscle mass, and create lifelong issues. An endocrinologist or primary care provider can help with these issues, assuming they understand the impact the eating disorder has made and do not use hormone therapy as the first step. You still have to be well nourished before hormones can help you. I have not seen any research on hormone use in gender transitions during an ED, but I would assume it should be put on pause for the same reasons given above.

For everyone of child-bearing age—just because your hormones are off or you don't have a period, does not mean that you cannot get pregnant or get someone pregnant. Please, use condoms if you are having sex. And "fun" fact—usually sex drive goes out the window with lack of nutrition. Your body is in survival mode, procreation is not a priority. Sex will be more enjoyable when you are eating enough. Seriously.

Weakened immune system

EDs, like any chronic illness, lower your immune response and make you more susceptible to getting sick. This means you will have a harder time fighting off illness, which can be fatal in some cases! This is primarily due to the lowered white blood cell counts (leukopenia). Eating enough food, eating a variety of food, and not pushing your body physically is your best defense against getting sick (along with washing your hands).

Make sure to get your flu shot (and other immunizations), get regular checkups with your medical provider, and PLEASE work on getting rid of your ED! The longer you are stuck in the disorder, the greater the likelihood for long-term health issues. You deserve so much better!

Substance abuse and ED

Eating disorders and substance use or abuse are closely related. Both are used as coping mechanisms for numbing or avoiding problems. Not only do about half of people with EDs abuse alcohol or drugs, but these behaviors can also flip-flop back and forth if underlying issues are not dealt with (usually in therapy).

The substances most abused by people with EDs (according to The National Center on Addiction and Substance Abuse in 2003): "caffeine, tobacco, alcohol, laxatives, emetics, diuretics, appetite suppressants, heroin, and cocaine." I will definitely agree with this list from what I have heard my college clients using (though no heroin yet, and let's keep it that way!).

Know that if you struggle with either an ED or substance abuse, you are at increased risk of developing the other, as many factors—most importantly, brain chemistry—are closely related. Unfortunately, most treatment centers either treat one or the other; not many are equipped to help with both simultaneously (detox and eating issues). Traditional plans have advised addressing the substance issues first, then the ED. However, if you can work on both at the same time, you have the greatest chance of health and recovery. One idea, if you cannot find a dual-residential center, is to get into detox and add therapy and RD support for the ED, even if it is virtual counseling.

When to go to urgent care (or emergency room)

I would like to preface this section with the note that I am not a doctor and have never worked in an emergency room/ED acute care. Please seek medical attention if you are concerned regardless of what I say here. You can always start with your primary care provider or urgent care if you are unsure.

- Resting heart rate below 40 (some will say 50, but usually the ER can't do much about it)
- Severe dehydration
- Haven't eaten (or haven't eaten more than a few hundred calories per day) for a week or longer.
- Fainting/blackouts
- Persistent chest pain

Main takeaways:

- Food is your medicine.
- Antidepressants (and other medications) might not be effective if you are malnourished.
- Only after you are eating enough food overall do we look at specific nutrients.

Take action:

When was the last time you had your hormone levels checked? It might be a good idea to ask your doctor or endocrinologist if you need some tests.

Do you struggle with anxiety or depression? Other mental illness? After reading the chapter, do you think your diet might be hurting your mental health? What easy change could you make?

Chapter 10

Your Amazing Body

"Love yourself first and everything else falls into line."

—Lucille Ball

D o you remember the last nice thing you said to your body?

Believe it or not, your body cares about you. It is your protector from the elements, your mode of transportation, the thing that carries around vital organs. In short, it is pretty dang miraculous! If you choose this book, I bet there is a good chance that you have (or had) a lot of hate, shame, and self-loathing about your own body.

But, seriously, think about all your body does for you.

It keeps you alive without you telling it to. Breathing, heart-beating, waste processing, food digesting into ENERGY (seriously, how cool is that!?!?!). You also have the strength to lift things, your hands are able to write, type and craft art. Your voice is able to speak and interact with people or sing and create music. The fact that your brain is able to process all of it, from reading the words on this page to understanding the meaning—that's amazing! You have skin and an immune system to help prevent illness, and you have eyes with which to see the beauty in every day. As you can tell, I am quite enamored with the human body.

The more I learn about the science of the body (or "physiology"), the more I am in awe of it. We can do so much harm to this sack of cells we live in, and yet it keeps on trucking. Wow.

I want you to think about what your body does for you and what it will be less likely to do if your eating disorder progresses. Creating peace between your mind and body takes work. Each time you say something nice to yourself, you make peace a little more possible.

Think about what our body does automatically

A lot of body processes happen without our thinking about it. Our lungs breathe and supply oxygen to all the cells in our body. We don't have to tell ourselves how to breathe, that's just something we do. We do it when we're asleep. We do it when we're awake.

Our heart beats. It pumps blood, nutrients, and oxygen all over our body so that we're able to carry out functions that keep us alive.

Our kidneys filter all the fluids in our body and take out minerals, leaving us with urine which our body excretes. And the fact that we have bladder and bowel control is pretty cool. How wonderful is the fact that our liver takes our nutrients through the blood and filters things that we don't want floating around in our bodies? It's our natural detoxifying system. We don't need to be on a crazy diet or cleanse for that to happen. Our body does it naturally.

Our stomach and intestines take food, any crazy kind of food, and break it down into single molecules. These molecules are taken through the intestines, the bloodstream, and transported to different cells for energy, for building our organs and all of our body tissues, to give us hormonal balance, for temperature regulation, to give us the hair on our head, and so much more! Our body is continuously doing all these crazy, amazing things.

We need to appreciate that we are also all designed to be unique and interesting individuals. If we all looked exactly the same, that would be a really boring world. It makes it more interesting that we all look a little different, that we can have different abilities, and we have different strengths and weaknesses. So, try not to be a carbon copy of anyone else because it's impossible.

Be your own unique you because that's what the world needs. There's no reason to be hating on yourself because you are awesome exactly as you are. As singer Demi Lovato put it so well, "What's wrong with being confident?"

Recovery is so worth it

"Recovery is so worth it. Your brilliant, miraculous body that has gone through so much in this eating disorder will be there for you as you finally learn how to nourish, rest, and be kind to it. Our bodies are built with amazing resiliency. Despite the damage that eating disorders cause, nearly all can be repaired with the simple realities of consistent nutrition, rest, and compassion. Have faith in your body, thank your body for sticking with you through it all, and trust that recovery is possible!"

—Jennifer L. Gaudiani, MD, CEDS, FAED
Founder & Director of the Gaudiani Clinic

Write a letter to a friend

Think of what your current standards of beauty are. In America and in a lot of developed countries, there is a thin ideal for women and a lean muscular ideal for men. I'm sure many other beauty standards also came up.

What if we didn't have to think about that?

How do you choose your friends? I would bet that you don't choose them based on how they look or what their weight is. You probably choose them because they're nice to you. You have similar interests. You can talk to them easily. They make you feel good about yourself. What are other reasons you have the friends you do?

Got that? Now, think about why your friends are friends with you. I'll tell you a little secret, it's not because of how you look. It's because you're a good friend to them, because you have similar interests, and because you make them feel good about themselves. Typically, it has nothing to do with how you actually look (though hygiene likely plays a role—bathe regularly, please).

For your homework today, I want you to take a little time and write a letter. I want this letter to be to your friend, or to your younger self. If you feel like sending it to that friend when you are done, go ahead and do it, it will make their day. If not, that's perfectly fine; it can be just for you.

Write about all the reasons why they are an amazing person and an amazing friend. I'd like you to leave looks out of it because that's not what it is about, is it? If you really think about it, it's not. Take that time to think about what makes them an awesome person. Why do you like spending time with them? If you're writing it to your younger self (and I highly encourage this), why are you awesome? Why do you not need to beat yourself up? What would you tell yourself three years ago?

Next, I would like you to write a love letter to your amazing body. This might be a harder one to write, but when you are feeling bad about your body, I think it is an important exercise. What does your body do for you? This is not a time to be humble. No one but you ever has to read it. Write this letter and read it again to yourself. Put it away for a while and pull it out in a few weeks and read it again.

When you pull that letter out again, take a look at what you wrote to your body. What do you need to do to honor and take better care of your body? Eat a more balanced diet? Eat enough? Spread your food out throughout the day instead of all at one sitting? Drink more water? Get more sleep? Envelop people in more hugs? How can you focus more on loving your body?

Health is about everything in moderation and balance. There are NO BAD FOODS. As someone who studied food and nutrition for eight years of higher education, plus my own study and work years between my bachelor's and master's degrees and beyond, I can tell you with 100 percent authority that unless a food is something you are truly allergic to or has bacteria that causes food poisoning (or is that weird part of pufferfish that is toxic), it will not kill you or do much damage.

Okay? Okay.

Think about how amazing the human body is—it can process a lot with minimal harm. Think about drug users and how long their bodies hold on. Think of all the super-processed food 90s kids like me ate with abandon— and, still, no issues here! Our bodies are extremely resilient!

Human resilience

A client of mine has put her body through so much in her eating disorder. Hundreds of laxatives, not eating for days, 10,000 Calorie binges. There is no reason she should still be alive, let alone thriving.

Her body (like yours) is incredible! Treat it with the love and respect it deserves. Seriously.

If writing the letter(s) came easily to you, take it a step further. Every time you look in the mirror, say something positive to yourself, something that you love about yourself, whether it's your appearance or your personality or something that your body does for you—take a minute every day to be thankful that you're alive and that you can move and do all the things that your amazing earth suit allows you to be able to do.

Helping a loved one

I would be remiss to not talk about how to help someone else you expect is experiencing disordered eating. Whether you have an ED or not, you can help someone else not have to stay stuck.

The most important thing you can do is just be a good friend. EDs are very isolating and make the person feel worthless. Sit with them, listen to them, and create a safe space. Judgment is a trust-killer. Once you have trust, here are some other things you can do to help.

1. Carefully confront them from a place of caring using "I statements". An "I statement" looks something like: "I am concerned that I never see you eat, despite how many times we all go out to dinner together. I am really worried about you." Or, "I see you spending an awful lot of time at the gym and I'm worried you are not letting your body have time to repair itself."

2. As a friend (or parent), you should NOT be the food police, but you can be the person who makes the difference between someone getting help or not. Be willing to help them seek out therapy or dietary appointments and go with them if they feel the need for support.

3. Don't talk about weight or body shape (yours or anyone else's), diets, being "bad" for eating something, or needing to "work it off." We *need* to change the norms around what is acceptable to talk about.

4. Model healthy eating habits. This is generally three meals a day, plus snacks as needed; or five to six "mini-meals" depending on your personal eating preferences. Food should encompass all food groups and be relatively balanced without being obsessive. For the general person consuming adequate calories, about 45 to 65 percent of calories should come from carbohydrates (grains, fruit, veggies, beans/legumes, nuts/seeds, dairy), 20 to 35 percent from fats (oils, avocado, nuts/seeds), and 10 to 35 percent from protein (meats, eggs, dairy, nuts/seeds, beans/legumes, soy). A normal, healthy diet provides space for what sounds good in the moment.

5. Help them deal with the underlying cause (if you can). Eating disorders are not about food. Food is used as a coping mechanism for another problem. Much like an alcoholic uses booze to numb the pain or check out of a situation, people with eating disorders use food to cope. Help them deal with the problem head on, help them to de-stress or take their mind off the problem in a healthy way (bowling, anyone?).

Some do's and don'ts on how to talk to someone with an (or suspected) ED, so as to not trigger them:

Do not...

- Tell them to "just eat something."
- Talk about your weight or body shape (especially negatively), or others'.
- Talk about a diet plan you follow or recommend a commercial diet plan. (If you're concerned about their eating habits, refer them to professionals who specialize in eating disorders.)
- Make weight or size an indicator of success (even a "positive" comment like, "you look great/healthy/slim" can be triggering).
- Take an ED lightly. Many patients will say, "My doctor didn't seem concerned/my doctor said I gained some weight, so I'm fine/my doctor told me I know what to do." Therefore, they do not believe they are "sick enough" to treat it as a problem. Any issues with food behaviors make them "sick enough" to get help.
- Make assumptions based on weight or physical appearance.

Do...

- Show them you are concerned using "I statements." For example: "I am concerned that you have lost a lot of weight in the last six months. I am afraid for your long-term health."
- Be compassionate. They are using food as a coping mechanism. They are probably stressed and overwhelmed, and possibly feeling unlovable.

- Explain what is going on in their body as they treat it the way they are, if it feels right (talk about long-term issues, what they could be losing, etc.).
- Get the family involved (if under 18, or willing to share with family or significant other). Teaching the whole family to work together in recovery is the best practice.

Main takeaways:

- Your body is resilient and does so much for you without you even having to think about it.
- Do's and don'ts for talking to someone you suspect has an ED.
- All foods fit in a healthy diet.

Take action:

Write a letter to a friend or your younger self.

Write a letter to your amazing body as it is today.

Be bold. Change the way you talk about yourself. Stop talking about looks or commenting on weight. Model healthy behaviors.

Chapter 11

You Got This!

"Forget all the reasons it won't work and believe the one reason why it will."

—Unknown

For some reason I've never understood, women and girls (especially, but all genders do) bond over commiserating about their "flawed" bodies. From junior high (and getting younger!) to old age, in popular media (*Mean Girls*, anyone?), putting down our own body somehow makes us "accepted" into the tribe.

How stupid!

Here's a novel idea: Don't put your body down to yourself or in front of others. Why would you hide your awesomeness? ED is such a manipulative b*tch, that your thoughts are twisted into believing that you are ugly/fat/[insert derogatory remark here]. I do believe you can change your beliefs about yourself. It's all about creating cognitive dissonance.

Cognitive dissonance (CD) is a term for when two conflicting thoughts, actions, or beliefs cause psychological stress, because they cannot coexist peacefully. Your brain wants to resolve the conflict by bringing one belief over to match the other. The good news is we can help decide what belief we keep through our actions. (In other words: fake it 'til you make it!) Here's what I did.

How my body confidence grew

Through the years preaching body love and confidence to not only my clients, but also friends and acquaintances, I found that my own self-talk became kinder with each season. CD wouldn't allow my personal beliefs to be opposite of my words and actions. It's one thing to understand the medical and mental aspects of an ED, but an entirely different understanding to believe full recovery is possible.

While working with people from all walks of life, all body types, abilities, and issues, I learned that it was so easy to find the beauty in others, and I needed to seek that out for myself. I couldn't see clients every day, tell them they are (truly) amazing and beautiful, and not start to hear it myself. This is exactly how cognitive dissonance works. My brain started to change and be shaped by my words and actions. I feel so much better about myself.

You can apply this to your own life by finding ways to create dissonance in your actions and thoughts. Tell people how awesome they are. Refuse to put down your body (even when everyone else is doing it). Tell yourself you look beautiful (or whatever word you would like to be called) in the mirror. Leave positive notes in public places, like bathroom mirrors. Wear the clothes you love, not the ones that you think make you look thinnest or whatever you are going for. Keep doing it and you will start to believe you are beautiful and worthy, just as you are.

When I was really struggling in college, food became a way to try to control a new environment that scared me. But I found that the more I avoided food, the more I thought about it—to the point where I couldn't be present in the other parts of my life. Dates were difficult as I fixated on where we were eating instead of the conversation. Schoolwork took more time than needed because I had food taking up valuable real estate in my mind as I studied. Despite the amount I exercised, I was definitely NOT the fittest I would be in my life.

Since making peace with food and my body, I have gone on to accomplish things that would have always been just out of reach while restricting. I ran a marathon (40 pounds above my lowest weight—which goes to show you that lower weight does not make you a better runner!). I have a real relationship and married a wonderful man. I own a business with which I am totally present and engaged. I can eat at any restaurant and eat what sounds good (rather than just the lowest-calorie option). I don't weigh myself and I am happier in my body than I ever was. I am a more confident performer and speaker. I have even auditioned for Broadway!

I'm telling you this not to brag, but to show you that YOU, too, can live a full life free of the negative thoughts that may currently run through your mind. Yes, anxiety and depression are still a part of my life (brain chemistry and all), and my food struggles are a part of my story, but they are only a PART of my story. There are a lot of chapters to go that have no room for food fear.

You don't have to go through this alone. The rat race to look a certain way or to avoid feelings is not what life is about. You can go live the incredible life you have imagined! **I give you permission to eat.**

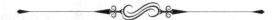

Thank you for taking the time to read this book. It tells me that you really value your health and well-being. At this point, do you know what you need to do next to support your recovery and self-esteem? Whatever your next step is, I hope you will continue to care for the one body and brain you get in this lifetime.

If you are interested in working more closely with me, please visit my professional website: www.NotYourAverageNutritionist. com

There you will find my services, videos, blog posts, and more support for your journey. I would love to hear from you!

You are so amazing!
Libby Parker, MS, RD

Acknowledgments

Thank you to so many people!

My husband who put up with the book taking over my life for many months, I love you. My writing coach and first editor, Laurence Currie-Clark; Morgan Gist MacDonald, and the entire team and community at Paper Raven Books who edited and managed my publishing. I couldn't have done it without you. My parents for all their love and support. All of my amazing clients who have given me the experience to write this book (and some who gave quotes to put in!). My friend and colleague Leslie Barber, who helped me fact-check some psychology parts. My friend and colleague Dr. Pamela Parker, who helped me fact-check some medical parts. My friends and colleagues who read my questionable first draft; and to all of the other wonderful supporters who made this book possible. I deeply thank you.

Appendix

First steps to recovery if you are stuck

For those of you putting off recovery from an eating disorder because of overwhelm, I want to give you some actionable steps in the form of a checklist to propel you forward. Here we go.

___ Get a physical with your primary care physician or a specialist. TELL THEM YOU HAVE AN EATING DISORDER. Explain what is going on. Most docs either don't ask the questions or are too rushed to do a thorough exam unless you tell them what is going on. Ask to have lab work done, and if your heart rate has slowed way down or is doing anything funky, ask for orthostatic vitals (blood pressure and heart rate; lying down, sitting, and standing, two to five minutes between each). KNOW YOUR NUMBERS (one exception is weight—you don't need to know your weight, and it is within your right to not know that number; just let them know before you get on the scale, and step on backward).

___ Tell someone what is going on. People who have social support from family and/or friends have much better outcomes. You don't need to shout it from a rooftop (unless you want to); just have someone cheering you on when it gets tough.

___ Find a professional. Assuming that you need outpatient-level care, find a licensed therapist (LMFT, LPCC, PsyD, or LCSW), a registered dietitian (RD or RDN), or both. Choosing someone who specializes in eating disorders is a big part of recovery and making peace with food and your body. The kind of professional you choose to start with depends on your comfort level. Typically, if you find one they can make referrals to the other. *(Shameless plug: I now do virtual counseling for clients in select US states. Email me if you are interested).* If you need higher level care (or don't know), they can help you look for treatment centers and get that process going if you haven't already.

Some great places to look for mental health professionals, RDs, doctors, and treatment programs if you don't have a treatment team set up yet:

https://www.edreferral.com/

www.psychologytoday.com

Just get started with those three steps, in any order.

It can be daunting, I know. Just take one step today.
Maybe it is setting up a doctor appointment.
Maybe it is searching for a short list of therapists to call.
Maybe it is telling your best friend what is going on with the only expectation being that they listen.

I'm already doing those things. What's next?

__ Add in some education. There are lots of great books, podcasts, blogs, and courses out there to assist with recovery.
Check out sites like:
https://www.notyouraveragenutritionist.com/resources.html
https://www.nationaleatingdisorders.org/blog
https://www.recoverywarriors.com/
https://www.edcatalogue.com/books/

__ Look for a support group. Through your dietitian or therapist, you might hear about support groups in your area. You can also search sites like: https://www.edreferral.com/easysearch.
My practice offers online recovery groups for people 18+ anywhere in the world. Check: https://www.notyouraveragenutritionist.com/group.html.

__ Be an advocate for body positivity. See if there is a local group of The Body Project near you or on campus, or just do your own version by not body shaming yourself or others. Encourage people around you to not talk themselves down or complain about wanting to lose weight. Talk to yourself like you would a friend. :)

The longer you put off recovery, the harder it gets.
But the good news is you can start anytime!
Whether it's been a month, six months, two years, or thirty, the time is NOW!
You can do this, I believe in you!

References

Chapter 1

Bermudez, O. (2013). Proceedings from iadep Meeting on Bio-Psycho Effects of Starvation, Exercise and Purging on Brain, & Serious Changes in Brain Psychology including Perspective on Patients. Santa Barbara, CA: iadep.

Burke, S. C., Cremeens, J., Vail-Smith, K., & Woolsey, C. L. (2010). Drunkorexia: Calorie restriction prior to alcohol consumption among college freshman. *Journal of Alcohol and Drug Education, 54*(2), 17-35.

Grodstein, F., Levine, R., Spencer, T., Colditz, G. A., & Stampfer, M. J. (1996). Three-year follow-up of participants in a commercial weight loss program: Can you keep it off? *Archives of Internal Medicine, 156*(12), 1302.

Neumark-Sztainer D., Haines, J., Wall, M., & Eisenberg, M. (2007). Why does dieting predict weight gain in adolescents? Findings from project EAT-II: a 5-year longitudinal study. *Journal of the American Dietetic Association, 107*(3), 448-455.

Neumark-Sztainer, D. (2005). *I'm, like, so fat!* New York: Guilford.

Chapter 2

Farrar, T. (2017, June). Stomach problems in anorexia recovery. [web log comment]. Retrieved from https://tabithafarrar.com/2017/06/anorexia-recovery-stomach-problems/.

Office of Disease Prevention and Health Promotion. (2015). *Dietary guidelines for Americans.* (Report No. 8). Retrieved from The Office of Disease Prevention and Health Promotion Website: https://health.gov/dietaryguidelines/2015/guidelines/.

Chapter 3

Golden, N. H., Schneider, M., & Wood, C. (2016). Preventing Obesity and Eating Disorders in Adolescents. *Pediatrics, 138*(3).

Herrin, M., & Larkin, M. (2012). *Nutrition Counselling in the Treatment of Eating Disorders. Abingdon: Routledge.*

Kennedy, D. O. (2016). B vitamins and the brain: Mechanisms, dose and efficacy—A review. *Nutrients, 8*(2), 68.

Thalheimer, J. C. (2016, October). Coconut oil. *Today's Dietitian*, *18*, 32.

The Whole Grains Council. (n.d.). Retrieved from https://wholegrainscouncil.org.

United States Department of Agriculture. (n.d.). USDA MyPlate. Retrieved from https://choosemyplate.gov.

Chapter 4

Fearmongering. (2010). In Oxford English dictionary online (3rd ed.), Retrieved from https://en.oxforddictionaries.com/definition/fearmongering.

National Institutes of Health, Office of Dietary Supplements. (2013). Frequently Asked Questions. Retrieved from https://ods.od.nih.gov/Health_Information/ODS_Frequently_Asked_Questions.aspx#Regulatory

Quackery. (2010). In Oxford English dictionary online (3rd ed.), Retrieved from https://en.oxforddictionaries.com/definition/quackery.

Chapter 5

Makhzoumi, S. H., Guarda, A. S., Schreyer, C. C., Reinblatt, S. P., Redgrave, G. W., & Coughlin, J. W. Chewing and spitting: A marker of psychopathology and behavioral severity in inpatients with an eating disorder. *Eating Behaviors*, *17*, 59-61.

Chapter 6

Beals, K. A., & Hill A. K. (2006). The prevalence of disordered eating, menstrual dysfunction, and low bone mineral density among US collegiate athletes. *International Journal of Sport Nutrition and Exercise Metabolism, 16*(1), 1-23.

Berczik, K., Szabo, A., Griffiths, M., Kurimay, T., Kun, B., Urban R., & Demetrovics, Z. (2012). Exercise addiction: Symptoms, diagnosis, epidemiology, and etiology. *Substance Use & Misuse, 47*, 403-417.

Bonci, L. (2004). *Sport nutrition for coaches*. Champaign, IL: Human Kinetics.

Byrne, S., & McLean, N. (2001). Eating disorders in athletes: A review of the literature. *Journal of Science and Medicine in Sport, 4*(2), 145-159.

Gaudiani, J. (2018). *Sick Enough*. Abingdon, UK: Routledge.

Golden, N. H., Schneider, M., & Wood, C. (2016). Preventing obesity and eating disorders in adolescents. *Pediatrics, 138*(3).

Greenleaf, C., Petrie, T. A., Carter, J., & Reel, J. J. (2009). Female collegiate athletes: Prevalence of eating disorders and disordered eating behaviors. *Journal of American College Health, 57*(5), 489-496.

Herrin, M., & Larkin, M. (2012). *Nutrition Counselling in the Treatment of Eating Disorders. 2ⁿᵈ Ed. Abingdon, UK: Routledge.*

Holtkamp, K., Hebebrand, J., & Herpetz-Dahlmann, B. (2004). The contribution of anxiety and food restriction on physical activity levels in acute anorexia nervosa. *The International Journal of Eating Disorders, 36*(2), 163-171.

Jankowski, C. (2012). Associations between disordered eating, menstrual dysfunction, and musculoskeletal injury among high school athletes. *Yearbook of Sports Medicine, 2012*, 394-395.

Lejoyeux, M., Avril, M., Richoux, C., Embouazza, H. & Nivoli, F. (2008). Prevalence of exercise dependence and other behavioral addictions among clients of a Parisian fitness room. *Comprehensive Psychiatry, 49*, 353-358.

Manley, R. O'Brien, K., & Samuels, S. (2008). Fitness instructors' recognition of eating disorders and attendant ethical/liability issues. *Eating Disorders: The Journal of Treatment & Prevention, 16*(2), 103-116.

Rubin, J. Knowledge, empowerment and conscious intention. Retrieved from https://jodirubin.wordpress.com.

Sundgot-Borgen, J., & Torstviet, M. K. (2004). Prevalence of eating disorders in elite athletes is higher than in the general population. *Clinical Journal of Sport Medicine, 14*(1), 25-32.

Thompson, R. A., & Sherman, R. T. (2010). *Eating disorders in sport*. New York, NY: Rutledge.

Chapter 8

Becker, A. E., Franko, D. L., Speck, A., & Herzog, D. B. (2003). Ethnicity and differential access to care for eating disorder symptoms. *International Journal of Eating Disorders,* *33*(2), 205-212.

Marques, L., Alegria, M., Becker, A. E., Chen, C., Fang, A., Chosak, A., & Diniz, J. B. (2011). Comparative prevalence, correlates of impairment, and service utilization for eating disorders across U.S. ethnic groups: Implications for reducing ethnic disparities in health care access for eating disorders. *The International Journal of Eating Disorders,* *44*(5), 412–420.

Wade, T. D., Keski-Rahkonen A., & Hudson J. (2011). *Epidemiology of eating disorders.* M. Tsuang & M. Tohen (Eds.). New York, NY: Wiley.

Chapter 9

Arcelus, J., Mitchell, A. J., Wales, J., & Nielsen, S. (2011). Mortality rates in patients with anorexia nervosa and other eating disorders. *Archives of General Psychiatry,* *68*(7), 724-731.

Deacon, G., Kettle, C., Hayes, D., Dennis, C., Tucci, J. (2017). Omega 3 polyunsaturated fatty acids and the treatment of depression. *Critical Reviews in Food Science and Nutrition,* *57*(1), 212-232.

Food for Thought: Substance Abuse and Eating Disorders. (2003, December). Retrieved from https://www. centeronaddiction.org/addiction-research/reports/food-thought-substance-abuse-and-eating-disorders.

Gaudiani, J. (2018). *Sick Enough*. Abingdon, UK: Routledge.

Godwin, K. (2018, November 5). Neurotransmitter production in relation to eating disorders [audio podcast]. Retrieved from https://www.listennotes.com/podcasts/ed-matters/episode-111-dr-katherine-fmTOjuGgd_b/.

Hosseinzadeh, M., Vafa, M., Esmaillzadeh, A., Feizi, A., Majdzadeh, R., Afshar, H., Keshteli A. H., Adibi, P. (2016). Empirically derived dietary patterns in relation to psychological disorders. *Public Health Nutrition, 19*(2), 204-217.

Huang, R., Wang, K., & Hu, J. (2016). Effect of probiotics on depression: A systematic review and meta-analysis of randomized controlled trials. *Nutrients, 8*(8), pii: E483.

Lang, U. E., Beglinger, C., Schweinfurth, N., Walter, M., & Borgwardt, S. (2015). Nutritional aspects of depression. *Cell Physiology and Biochemistry, 37*(3), 1029-1043.

Lim, S. Y., Kim, E. J., Kim, A., Lee, H, J., Choi, H. J., & Yang, S. J. (2016). Nutritional factors affecting mental health. *Clinical Nutrition Research, 5*(3), 143-152.

Marx, W., Moseley, G., Berk, M., & Jacka, F. (2017). Nutritional psychiatry: The present state of the evidence. *Proceedings of the Nutritional Society, 76*(4), 427-436.

Opie, R. S., Itsiopoulos, C., Parletta, N., Sanchez-Villegas, A., Akbaraly, T. N., Ruusunen, A., & Jacka, F. N. (2017). Dietary recommendations for the prevention of depression. *Nutritional Neuroscience, 20*(3), 161-171.

Papadopoulos, F. C., Ekbom, A., Brandt, L., & Ekselius, L. (2008). Excess mortality, causes of death and prognostic factors in anorexia nervosa. *The British Journal of Psychiatry, 194*(1), 10-17.

Pinto-Sanchez, M., Hall, G. B., Ghajar, K., Nardelli, A., Bolino, C., Lau, J. T., . . .Bercik, P. (2017). Probiotic Bifidobacterium longum NCC3001 reduces depression scores and alters brain activity: A pilot study in patients with irritable bowel syndrome. *Gastroenterology, 153*(2), 448-459.

The National Center on Addiction and Substance Abuse (CASA) at Columbia University. Food for Thought: Substance Abuse and Eating Disorders. The National Center on Addiction and Substance Abuse (CASA) Columbia University; New York: 2003.

Author Bio

Libby Parker, MS, RD

Libby is a Registered Dietitian and owner of Not Your Average Nutritionist, LLC, an outpatient practice for eating disorder recovery. She lives in California with her husband (a fantastic nurse) and two dogs, and loves performing in musical theatre every chance she gets. *Permission To Eat* is her first book, of (she hopes) many.

Connect with Libby on Facebook or Instagram @DietitianLibby